Work and the Eye

Work and the Eye

Rachel V. North

Department of Optometry and Vision Sciences
University of Wales College of Cardiff

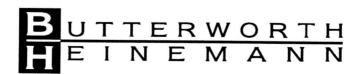

Butterworth-Heinemann
Linacre House, Jordan Hill, Oxford OX2 8DP
225 Wildwood Avenue, Woburn, MA 01801-2041
A division of Reed Educational and Professional Publishing Ltd

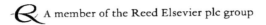 A member of the Reed Elsevier plc group

OXFORD   BOSTON   JOHANNESBURG
MELBOURNE   NEW DELHI   SINGAPORE

First published by Oxford University Press 1993
Paperback edition 1998

British Library Cataloguing in Publication Data
A catalogue record for this book is availaboe from the British Library

Library of Congress Cataloguing in Publication Data
North, Rachel V.
    Work and the eye/Rachel V. North
    1. Optometry   2. Industrial hygiene   3. Eye-
    wounds and injuries - Prevention
    I. Title   II. Series
    RE952.N67   1993   617'.7'15-dc20   92-22606

ISBN 0 7506 4045 6

Printed in Hong Kong

Preface

For the past 10 years I have taught the course of Occupational Optometry to undergraduate students. It is a course that includes many different topics and there has not been a textbook available covering the entire course that could be recommended to students. Therefore, I embarked on the project of writing this textbook in an attempt to provide a single source of information for those concerned with the field of occupational optometry. The ability to perform a visual task efficiently and safely depends on the visual capabilities of the person and the visibility of the task. One of the aims of this book is to identify some of the potential visual problems in carrying out a given task and offer guidance to enable visual performance to be maximized. For example, many people will have experienced eye strain when working with a visual display unit. This may be due either to uncorrected vision or to factors of poor work station design, such as an incorrect level of lighting or the presence of glare sources. This textbook also discusses the visual standards required for certain tasks and methods of vision screening available. Ocular hazards and the injuries that may result from unintentional exposure are also described. From studies investigating the incidence and causes of ocular injuries it appears that most are preventable, especially by the provision and use of the correct type of eye-protector. The various types of eye-protectors available are discussed and details are given regarding eye-protection programmes. Also outlined are the current standards, codes, and regulations relating to eye-protection, including the legal duties of both employers and employees.

It is hoped that this textbook will be of interest to undergraduate and practising optometrists, but also to health and safety officers, occupational hygienists, occupational nurses, and others involved in eye care.

Cardiff   R.V.N.
April 1993

Acknowledgements

I would like to express my sincere thanks to all those who have given assistance in the writing of this book. In particular, I am indebted to John Grundy, BSc, FBCO, and Professor Millodot, OD, PhD, FAAO, FBCO, for their comments, suggestions, and corrections of the manuscript and above all for their encouragement. I also wish to thank the AOP, HMSO, and BSI for their assistance and permission to copy sections of their standards and regulations and the Chartered Institution of Building Services, the Electricity Association Services Ltd, and Thorn Lighting for the many tables and figures extracted from their publications.

Contents

1. Visual performance

There are many varied and complex types of work in industry today. Any professional engaged to advise on visual performance would need, in the first instance, to visit the place of work to gain a full understanding of the task(s) and obtain a precise knowledge of its demand(s) upon the employee. The goal is to minimize stress on the visual system, which will result in an efficient and safe visual performance. In addition to the assessment of the work place and the tasks involved, an assessment of individual capabilities is required to determine whether the visual abilities match the visual requirements of the job. If not, one of two things can happen: (i) changes can be made to the work place; or (ii) direct assistance can be given to the employee, for example, in the form of spectacles or magnifiers.

The ability to perform most tasks depends on many visual and non-visual variables, and the factors that influence the visual performance can be listed as follows:

(1) the visual capability of the individual;
(2) the visibility of the task;
(3) psychological and general physiological factors.

It is not within the scope of this text to deal with the third group of factors in depth, although psychological and general physiological factors, such as motivation, intelligence, general health, etc. should not be forgotten, because they can all influence the visual performance. This chapter will deal with the first two variables—visual capabilities and the visibility of the task.

Visual capabilities

A knowledge of the capabilities and limits of the visual system is essential so that tasks can be designed to allow maximum performance and a minimum number of errors. A task that requires the visual system to operate at its limit may cause general stress, asthenopia, and decreased performance and efficiency. Far too often insufficient attention is given to determining the visual capabilities of a person and to ensuring that he or she is capable of seeing adequately in relation to the demands of a particular task.

The functions of the visual system can be divided into four broad groups:

(1) detection;
(2) recognition;
(3) colour discrimination;
(4) depth perception.

The functions and factors that influence the above visual parameters have been described thoroughly in many books (see Further reading) and they are the main sources used to compile this chapter.

Detection

The functions involved in the detection of objects include the following:

(1) visual field;
(2) head and eye movements;
(3) light perception;
(4) visual adaptation;
(5) flicker frequency;
(6) contrast sensitivity.

Visual field

The stationary eye can detect a visual stimulus within an area extending 60 degrees superiorly, 70 degrees inferiorly, 95 degrees temporally, and 60 degrees nasally. The total horizontal visual field extends to 190 degrees; 145 degrees being the monocular visual field and with a 120 degree binocular overlap (Weston 1962). The sensitivity of the retina to a stimulus varies; the retina is least sensitive at the periphery and most sensitive at the fovea.

Detection of a visual stimulus will depend on its size, distance, colour, and on the background illumination. Different occupations make different demands on the visual field. Some tasks, such as VDU work, make little demand on the peripheral visual field but a lot on the central visual field. Other tasks, such as driving or flying, where safety is a major concern, require full visual fields.

Individuals with monocular vision are at a disadvantage because, not only do they have a reduced visual field, but they do not have the binocular overlap to compensate for the blind spot. Consequently they have an absolute scotoma within their field of view. It is important to allow for the length of time that an individual has been monocular, and therefore the time that they have had to adapt to the loss of visual field, as well as to the loss of stereopsis. For example, in Sweden, a person who has lost the vision in one eye is barred from driving for 1 year, to allow time for adaptation.

Age influences the extent of visual field—the lateral visual field declines after the age of 35 years (Burg 1968). The restriction of the field is thought to be partly due to senile enophthalmos—a sinking of the globe within the orbit. Drance et al. (1967) also found an age-related loss of visual field, particularly in the superior field. They found a decrease in sensitivity of 1 dB per decade averaged over the total visual field. Haas *et al.* (1986) found that age appeared to influence the sensitivity of the upper half of the visual field to a greater extent than the lower half; the periphery and the centre were found to be more affected than the pericentric area. The sensitivity was found to decrease, on average, by 0.58 dB per decade.

Visual fields may be unintentionally restricted by: (i) a heavy library— type of spectacle frame; (ii) opaque side shields on safety spectacles; or (iii) the lens type. Any person requiring full visual fields for an occupation/task should be provided with spectacle frames and lenses of a type that least restricts the field of view.

Head and eye movement

Detection ability is enhanced by both head and eye movements. Eye movements are controlled by four neurological systems (Robinson 1968):

(1) saccadic;

(2) smooth pursuit;

(3) vestibular;

(4) vergence.

The visual environment may be sampled by fast conjugate eye movements (400–600 degrees/s) known as saccades, which locate an object of interest on the fovea. Fixation of the object is maintained by slow pursuit movements for objects that are moving at less than 45 degrees/s. Corrective saccades are required to follow objects moving at speeds greater than 45 degrees/s. The stabilization of the eyes with regard to the environment during head and body movements is the function of the vestibular system. The vergence system allows accurate fixation of the object of regard located at any distance in the visual field, and hence it acts as a range-finding system, which can interact with the other systems.

The extent of the horizontal and vertical eye movements is in the range of 45–50 degrees either side of the primary position, but head movements generally occur when the eye movement exceeds 15 degrees. Therefore a person reading at a desk will lower their head rather than depress the eyes (Weston 1962).

Tasks requiring frequent changes in direction of gaze can be visually fatiguing and cause discomfort. This is most likely to occur when the eyes are near the limit of their range. In addition, there will be different amounts of accommodation and convergence required for different viewing distances. Visual discomfort is therefore more likely to occur in people with poor convergence and fusion when viewing near tasks. A presbyopic worker wearing a bifocal prescription may have to adopt an unnatural head posture when the viewing distance is either at or above eye level. An example would be a pilot's instrument panel, some of which is above head level and require the head to be tilted back to an unnatural angle to see through the near vision segment of the bifocal. Care should therefore be taken when prescribing for the presbyope; the type of lens and the height and size of the near addition segment must be appropriate for the task.

Light perception and visual adaptation

The visual system can operate over a very large range of luminances due to the actions of the photoreceptors—the rods and cones. At luminances below 10^{-6} cd/m^2 there is insufficient light for the visual system to operate. The rods function at luminance levels between 10^{-6} and 10^{-3} cd/m^2, which is referred to as scotopic vision. An intermediate state exists where both the rods and cones operate at levels between 10^{-3} and 3 cd/m^2; this is mesopic vision. Above luminances of 3 cd/m^2 the rods are completely saturated and only the cones function; this is photopic vision (Boyce 1981).

The spectral responses of the rods and cones are different; the peak sensitivity for cones occurs at 555 nm and that for rods at 505 nm. The spectral response of the eye will change as luminance shifts from scotopic to photopic conditions. This is known as the Purkinje shift. Colours are not visible under scotopic conditions, as only the rods are functioning. Colour is gradually recognized as the luminance level is increased, until full colour vision is acquired under photopic conditions.

ABSOLUTE THRESHOLD

The absolute threshold represents the smallest amount of light that gives rise to a visual sensation. The threshold will depend on the spectral nature of the light, which increases from white to red to violet (Gunkel and Gouras 1963). The absolute threshold is found to increase with age. This is thought to be partly due to senile miosis and greater absorption of the crystalline lens, which reduce the amount of light reaching the retina. The latter is proportional of the pupil area. Therefore as the pupil size decreases with age, the amount of light reaching the retina will also decrease. There will also be a larger absorption of blue light within the crystalline lens as it yellows with age, resulting in a more marked increase in the blue light threshold when compared to other wavelengths.

DARK ADAPTATION

Retinal sensitivity can increase by 100 000 times after half an hour in a dark room. This remarkable sensitivity to the detection of light is called dark adaptation, i.e. change in absolute threshold with time (Fig. 1.1). The process has three phases:

1. A rapid phase involving neural mechanisms.
2. A medium time phase of adjustment of the pupil size.
3. A slow phase due to the regeneration of the photosensitive pigments.

The regeneration of the cone pigments is faster than that of the rods, being approximately 2 min and 8 min, respectively. Adaptation is rapid if the initial and final adaptation luminances are both in the photopic range, as only the cones are involved. If the initial luminance level is in the scotopic range then adaptation takes longer, as it involves pigment regeneration of both the rods and cones.

The adaptation process is influenced by such factors as size and colour of the adapting and test fields, initial and final luminance of the test field, and the area of retina stimulated.

Age will also influence the dark adaptation process. The dark adaptation

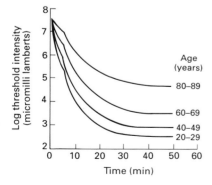

Fig. 1.1 Dark adaptation as a function of age. The threshold intensity is measured in micromillilamberts (after McFarland *et al.* 1960).

curves for increasing ages lie parallel to one another, and the threshold increases; this is shown in Figure 1.1. The dark adaptation is slower with age and the same level of sensitivity is not achieved. The intensity of the light stimulus has to be doubled for each 13 years of age (Domey and McFarland 1961). It is because of this reduced dark adaptation ability that many elderly drivers feel unsafe driving at night.

DIFFERENTIAL THRESHOLD

When the eye has adapted to a new luminance level it can then function to distinguish or detect objects. The ability of the eye to detect a stimulus can be described in terms of the smallest increment of luminance (ΔI) that can be detected from a uniform background luminance (I). This is known as the differential threshold and ΔI is usually directly proportional to I ($\Delta I / I = 1/100$); this is the Fechner Law (Davson 1990). Once again, other factors that will influence the differential threshold include size and colour of the object, state of adaptation of the eye, and duration of exposure. The differential threshold also increases with age, as does the effect of glare upon the differential threshold (Wolf 1960). This is thought to be partly due to the scattering of light by the ocular media, which occurs with age (Weale 1961).

The ability to see well at low levels of illumination is not a common requirement of many occupations. However it is particularly important in tasks such as driving, flying or sailing at night, or photographic dark-room work.

Flicker frequency

If the frequency of a flickering light is steadily increased a point will be reached where the light appears to be steady. The frequency at which the flicker ceases, is known as the critical fusion frequency (CFF). It can be taken as a measure of the temporal resolving power of the visual system. The CFF depends on many factors, including size, colour, and luminance of the stimulus; the area of retina being stimulated; and the duration of the flashes. The CFF increases with the size and luminance of the flickering stimulus and it is generally higher in the peripheral than in the central retinal regions. Fluorescent lights and movie films flicker but we are unaware of it, because they are designed to flicker at a rate above the CFF. Some reports suggest a decrease in the CFF after 50 years of age. Hence lights that are seen to be flickering by a younger person may be seen as fused/steady by an older person (Brozek and Keys 1945; Weale 1965). This is believed to be partly due to an increase in the persistence of stimuli in the nervous system with age (Axelrod 1963; Botwinick 1978).

Contrast sensitivity

Contrast sensitivity is the ability to detect border contrast. It is the reciprocal of the minimum perceptible contrast. It is an evaluation of the detection of objects in tests usually presented as sinusoidal gratings, of varying spatial frequencies, and of variable contrast. The acuity for gratings is specified by spatial frequency in cycles/degree. When the spatial frequency is plotted as a function of the contrast between the lines and

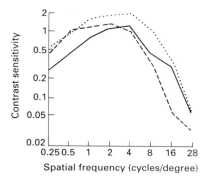

Fig. 1.2 Contrast sensitivity functions for different age groups (———) 8–15 years, (. . . . .) 18–39 years and (- - - - -) 45–66 years. The contrast sensitivity is the reciprocal of the contrast threshold. Contrast = $L_{max} - L_{min}/L_{max} + L_{min}$, where L_{max} and L_{min} are the maximum and minimum luminances (cd/m^2) in the grating display, respectively (after Arundale 1978; reproduced by kind permission of the British Medical Association).

spaces forming the grating, the plot is termed the contrast sensitivity function. It is generally accepted that the contrast sensitivity improves with age up to the thirties. Figure 1.2 shows that the 18–39-year-old group is optimal at all frequencies. The 45–66-year-old group is similar up to 0.5 cycles per degree and then the contrast sensitivity decreases especially in the 4–20 cycles/degree range (Arundale 1978). If the contrast sensitivity is measured as a function of retinal illumination the sensitivity difference is reduced but not eliminated. (A visual acuity of 6/6 is equivalent to 30 cycles per degree.) Binocular thresholds are lower than monocular ones and this is most marked for high frequencies. As the environment and the tasks performed within it are not composed of high contrast objects alone, but also of those of medium and low contrast, it is often suggested that contrast sensitivity is a better assessment of a person's visual capabilities to perform such tasks as driving.

Recognition

Static acuity

Static visual acuity is the capacity for seeing distinctly the details of a stationary object. Quantitatively, it is represented in two ways: (i) as the reciprocal of the minimum angle of resolution, in minutes of arc; and (ii) as the Snellen fraction.

The usual method of specifying visual acuity (VA) is by using letters, which are expressed as a Snellen fraction. The Snellen letter is constructed on an equal-sided grid, so that each limb width is one-fifth of the letter height. The letter size is expressed as a Snellen fraction in the form 6/6, 6/9, 6/12, etc., where the numerator is the test distance in metres and the denominator is the distance at which the letter subtends 5 min of arc. Normal visual acuity by this notation is 6/6, which means that a letter of 5 min of arc with a limb separation of 1 min of arc can be resolved at 6 m.

There are numerous factors—physical, physiological, and psychological—which can influence the ability of the visual system to see details. These can be listed as follows: luminance, contrast, spectral nature of light, size and intensity of surrounding field, region of retina stimulated, distance and size of object, time available to see object, glare, foggy/steamy atmosphere, refractive error, pupil size, age, attention, IQ, boredom, ability to interpret blurred images, general health, and emotional state (Riggs 1965; Westheimer 1987). Some of the major factors will now be discussed.

DISTANCE OF THE TASK

Naturally, the distance of the task from the observer and the size of the detail of the task affect the retinal image size, and hence the visual acuity required to distinguish it. The distance of the task also determines the level of accommodation and convergence and the degree of uncorrected refractive error or phoria that may be tolerated. Working distances may be classified as: far (> 2 m), intermediate-to-near (< 2 m and > 30 cm), and very near (< 30 cm) (Grundy 1988). Examples of tasks involving far working distances include driving a vehicle and flying an airplane;

intermediate-to-near tasks include secretarial work, VDU operating, and lathe operating; and very near tasks include sewing, micro-electronics assembly work, and watch repairing.

The amount of accommodation decreases with age, and generally, after their mid-forties workers require a spectacle prescription to focus near objects clearly and comfortably. As the range of accommodation reduces with age, the range of clear vision through the various near vision additions becomes smaller. Table 1.1 shows the range of clear vision obtainable by the emmetrope (or ametrope with corrected distance vision) and through the various additions according to the patient's usable accommodation (Grundy 1987). It must be remembered that the table shows the average amount of accommodation for the various ages and that there is natural variation between individuals, and that accommodation is also influenced by general health and certain medications. The amount of accommodation that can be exerted for a prolonged period of time is one-half the total accommodation available (Millodot and Millodot 1989) and the table takes this into account when stating the amount of usable accommodation. It can be used to indicate the most effective combination of powers of prescriptions to provide clear vision at all the required distances, and to show that it is not always possible to fulfil the needs of the presbyope with a 'normal' prescription. For example, consider the visual requirements of a 45 year-old VDU operator who needs to see the VDU screen at 70 cm and the documents at 35 cm. The amplitude of accommodation is $+3.50$ dioptres (D) for a 45-year-old and the amount that can be exerted for a prolonged period of time is half that, i.e. $+1.75$ D. Inspection of the 'age' column of Table 1.1 shows that $+1.25$ D addition will give clear vision from 33.33 to 80 cm, and so the visual requirements will be satisfied. If, however, the operator is older, e.g. 55 years old, it is not possible to view the required distances with a single addition. The 55-year-old will have $+1.50$ D of accommodation, of which $+0.75$ D is usable. To focus the screen at 70 cm an addition of $+0.75$ or $+1.00$ D could be used, but the document—at 35 cm—will not be seen clearly with either. To focus at 35 cm an addition of $+2.25$ D is required, and therefore a lens that incorporates these powers must be selected.

It must be remembered that the ageing eye takes longer to relax accommodation when looking from near to far than from far to near. This usually gives rise to complaints of temporary blurred vision when looking from a near task to some objects of attention in the distance. Also, if the working distance is very close, base in prism may be required to take the strain off the convergence system.

Size of task

The size of the critical detail of the task needs to be taken into account so that the angle subtended at the eye, and hence the visual acuity necessary to perform the task comfortably and efficiently can be calculated. The retinal image size of any object is inversely proportional to its distance from the eye. Therefore objects may differ greatly in physical dimensions but form similar retinal image size due to the fact that they are viewed at different distances. So, whilst the visual acuity may be the same, the

Table 1.1 Range of clear vision (cm) with reading prescriptions (reproduced by kind permission of J.W. Grundy and *Optometry Today* 1987)

Age (years)	40	42	45	48	50	52	55	60	65
Amplitude of accommodation (D)	4.50	4.00	3.50	3.00	2.50	2.00	1.50	1.00	0.50
Usable accommodation (D)	2.25	2.00	1.75	1.50	1.25	1.00	0.75	0.50	0.25

Range of clear vision (cm)

Power of add (D)		40	42	45	48	50	52	55	60	65
Plano		44.4	50.0	57.1	66.6	80.0	100.0	133.3	200.0	400.0
		Infinity	Infinity	Infinity	Infinity	Infinity	Infinity	Infinity	Infinity	Infinity
+0.50		36.4	40.0	44.4	50.0	57.1	66.7	80.0	100.0	133.3
		200.0	200.0	200.0	200.0	200.0	200.0	200.0	200.0	200.0
+0.75		33.3	36.4	40.0	44.4	50.0	57.1	66.7	80.0	100.0
		133.3	133.3	133.3	133.3	133.3	133.3	133.3	133.3	133.3
+1.00		30.8	33.3	36.4	40.0	44.4	50.0	57.1	66.7	80.0
		100.0	100.0	100.0	100.0	100.0	100.0	100.0	100.0	100.0
+1.25		28.6	30.8	33.3	36.4	40.0	44.4	50.0	57.1	66.7
		80.0	80.0	80.0	80.0	80.0	80.0	80.0	80.0	80.0
+1.50		26.7	28.6	30.8	33.3	36.4	40.0	44.4	50.0	57.1
		66.7	66.7	66.7	66.7	66.7	66.7	66.7	66.7	66.7

+1.75	25.0 / 57.1	26.7 / 57.1	28.6 / 57.1	30.8 / 57.1	33.3 / 57.1	36.4 / 57.1	40.0 / 57.1	44.4 / 57.1	50.0 / 57.1
+2.00	23.5 / 50.0	25.0 / 50.0	26.7 / 50.0	28.6 / 50.0	30.8 / 50.0	33.3 / 50.0	36.4 / 50.0	40.0 / 50.0	44.4 / 50.0
+2.25	22.2 / 44.4	23.5 / 44.4	25.0 / 44.4	26.7 / 44.4	28.6 / 44.4	30.0 / 44.4	33.3 / 44.4	36.4 / 44.4	40.0 / 44.4
+2.50	21.1 / 40.0	22.2 / 40.0	23.5 / 40.0	25.0 / 40.0	26.7 / 40.0	28.6 / 40.0	30.8 / 40.0	33.3 / 40.0	36.4 / 40.0
+2.75	20.0 / 36.4	21.1 / 36.4	22.2 / 36.4	23.5 / 36.4	25.0 / 36.4	26.7 / 36.4	28.6 / 36.4	30.8 / 36.4	33.3 / 36.4
+3.00	19.1 / 33.3	20.0 / 33.3	21.1 / 33.3	22.2 / 33.3	23.5 / 33.3	25.0 / 33.3	26.7 / 33.3	28.6 / 33.3	30.8 / 33.3
+3.25	18.2 / 30.8	19.1 / 30.8	20.0 / 30.8	21.1 / 30.8	22.2 / 30.8	23.5 / 30.8	25.0 / 30.8	26.7 / 30.8	28.6 / 30.8
+3.50	17.4 / 28.6	18.2 / 28.6	19.1 / 28.6	20.0 / 28.6	21.1 / 28.6	22.2 / 28.6	23.5 / 28.6	25.0 / 28.6	26.7 / 28.6

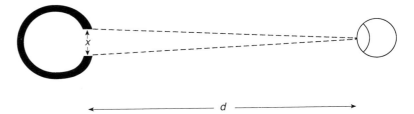

Fig. 1.3 Angular size of the criticial detail (*d*, working distance; *x*, size of critical detail).

demands made upon accommodation and convergence may be different. A very small object may have to be placed very close for the detail to be large enough to be resolved, but this will require good accommodation and convergence.

The angle subtended at the eye, and hence the visual acuity required, can be calculated mathematically (see Fig. 1.3):

$$\text{Tan visual angle} = \frac{\text{size of critical detail}}{\text{working distance}} \tag{1.1}$$

or graphically using a Nomogram (see Fig. 2.1). Table 1.2 shows the optimum visual acuity required for the different visual angles (Grundy 1988). The visual acuity necessary should be approximately twice that of the minimum calculated (Grundy 1981) so that the individual is not working at their limit. If the visual angle is less than 3 min of arc then it may be worthwhile considering magnification to increase the angular subtense of the task at the eye. This is particularly useful in the electronics industry. Magnification may be provided by hand- or stand-magnifiers,

Table 1.2 Visual acuity and angular size of critical detail (reproduced by kind permission of J.W. Grundy and Butterworth–Heinemann (Oxford) Ltd 1988)

	Angular size of critical detail (minutes of arc)	Minimum VA required	Optimum VA required	
Large	10.0	6/60	6/30	N20
Medium	6.0	6/36	6/18	N12
Small	3.0	6/18	6/9	N6
Very small	1.5	6/9	6/4.5	N3
Minute	0.75	6/4.5	Magnification + good VA required	

The near point equivalents refer to a viewing distance of 40 cm.
VA, visual acuity.

which may have built-in illumination, monocular or binocular loupes, or more complicated devices, such as microscopes, telescopes, and binoculars for distant objects or projection devices.

LUMINANCE AND CONTRAST
Two major factors that influence visual acuity are luminance and contrast. The influence of luminance upon visual acuity is shown in Figure 1.4. The capacity of the visual system to resolve details increases with increasing luminance, although there is a level beyond which visual acuity does not increase: in fact it may diminish due to disability glare. Contrast has a maximal effect on visual acuity at low levels of illumination but a minimal effect at high levels.

AGE
There is a small decline in visual acuity with age. The general causes are cataract, macular degeneration, and glaucoma, particularly in the over-70 age group (Grey *et al.* 1989). However, visual acuity is not normally affected during the working life-time (Fig. 1.5).

TIME AVAILABLE
The time available to view the letters, etc. will influence the visual acuity measured. It has been estimated that a person can transmit up to 10 bits/s (a bit is a unit of information) of visually displayed information. This is a very small amount of information, when it is estimated that the human sensory system has a capacity to transmit millions of bits/s. Therefore it is not the input of the visual system that limits the visual performance but the processing, decision-making, and motor output. Letters can usually be recognized in under a second and, obviously, the better the illumination and the larger the letter, the faster the recognition time.

REFRACTIVE ERROR
It is generally agreed that in early childhood the normal eye is hyperopic. Later, the refraction shifts towards emmetropia until the early twenties.

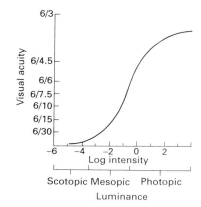

Fig. 1.4 The relationship between visual acuity and luminance (measured in millilamberts). (Königs data replotted by Hecht 1934).

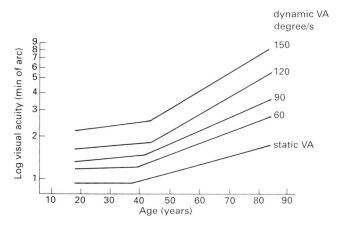

Fig. 1.5 Static and dynamic visual acuities as a function of age (after Hills 1975; reproduced by kind permission of the Transport and Road Research Laboratory).

The refraction then stays relatively stable until the forties, when a hypermetropic shift may occur. In the later years there may be a myopic shift, known as index myopia, which occurs due to nuclear sclerosis of the crystalline lens. The astigmatism also changes with age. Most children have astigmatism 'with the rule', i.e. the vertical meridian of the cornea is steeper than the horizontal. This changes throughout life so that the majority of people in later life show 'against the rule' astigmatism, i.e. the horizontal meridian of the cornea is steeper than the vertical. The greatest change in astigmatism occurs between the ages of 30 and 50 years (Weale 1963).

An ametropic person generally requires a spectacle prescription. However, for certain tasks it may be beneficial to leave the eyes uncorrected. For example, uncorrected myopes have been found to be far more efficient at their hosiery task than hyperopes, as they did not have to accommodate to see the task detail. It has been estimated that one-third of employees have uncorrected or insufficiently corrected refractive errors that affect visual acuity, efficiency, and comfort (Ungar 1971). Often, it is the presbyopic worker whose visual efficiency is reduced, as they require a near vision addition that they fail to have updated regularly.

VERNIER ACUITY

The type of visual acuity discussed so far has been form acuity—the ability to discriminate between two small parts of an object. However, in some occupations line detail is required, for example, the use of micrometers or precision gauges requires the discrimination of a break in contour or alignment, i.e. vernier acuity. The visual system is extremely sensitive to these details and it is approximately one-twentieth of the corresponding angle for details to be resolved in form acuity (Grundy 1988). If the form acuity for a certain distance is known then it is relatively easy to calculate the equivalent visual angle for vernier acuity and the actual size that may be resolved, and vice versa. Misalignments of segments of a divided line of approximately 3 s of arc can be detected at moderately high levels of illumination, whereas the minimum angle of resolution is between 30–60 s of arc (Westheimer 1987).

Dynamic visual acuity

The visual system can not only detect moving objects but can also discriminate and identify the object. Dynamic (kinetic) visual acuity is the term used to define the acuity based on a moving target. The discrimination of detail of a moving object depends upon the ability of the eyes to remain fixated on it. At slow speeds the acuity is nearly the same as for static tests but as the speed is increased the dynamic visual acuity decreases. Head movements are required for target speeds of above 60 degrees/s otherwise there is a marked drop in acuity. Dynamic visual acuity is not directly related to static visual acuity. It is influenced by target angular velocity, target exposure time, luminance, contrast, extent of visual field, paramacular visual acuity, method of tracking—head and eye movements, reaction time, learning factors, and fatigue (Ludvigh and Miller 1958; Fergenson and Suzansky 1973). A progressive decline in dynamic visual acuity has been shown to occur with age (see Fig. 1.5;

Burg 1966, Reading 1968). Younger people are better at tracking fast moving objects than older. This is partly due to an increase in the latent period of onset of a following eye movement as age increases (Sharpe and Sylvester 1978; Spooner *et al.* 1980).

Dynamic visual acuity is believed to be a more reliable measure of a person's ability to perform such tasks as driving or inspection tasks on a conveyor belt than the conventional static test.

Colour discrimination

Under photopic conditions the human visual system has a highly developed colour sense. The sensation of colour is subjective but it can be analysed in terms of three attributes: (i) hue; (ii) saturation; and (iii) luminous intensity. It has been estimated that a person with normal colour vision can discriminate millions of detectably different colours. These estimates are based upon comparison of colours placed adjacent to one another, but for absolute judgements only about 30 colours can be identified reliably (Bishop and Crook 1961). The fine colour discrimination of the visual system is such that it can discriminate most colours whose wavelengths differ by less than 5 nanometres (nm).

Colour discrimination depends upon:

(1) state of adaptation of retina;

(2) region of retina stimulated;

(3) simultaneous contrast;

(4) successive contrast.

Colour vision extends 20–30 degrees from the fovea. Beyond this the ability to discern colour is lost, as is the case in scotopic conditions. The ability to discriminate a colour from its background will be influenced greatly by the respective colours. This is especially the case when the luminance contrast between the object and its background is very small, so that colour contrast is the only method of discrimination. The colour of an object can also be perceived differently depending on the colour of the background. This is known as *simultaneous contrast*, when the colour of the object tends towards the complementary colour of the background. For example a grey spot viewed against a red background will appear greenish. Similarly, a person may complain of coloured after-images due to prior exposure to another colour. This is known as *successive contrast*, where the after-image tends towards the complementary colour of the initial exposure. For example, after viewing an ocular fundus through a red-free filter (i.e. a green filter) a reddish after image is seen.

Colour defective vision may be congenital or acquired. The most common type is congenital, which affects more men (8 per cent) than women (0.5 per cent) (Voke 1980). Three types of defective colour vision are usually recognized: (i) anomalous trichromatism; (ii) dichromatism; and (iii) monochromatism. The last is total colour blindness, in which there is a perception of luminance but not of colour. Anomalous trichromatism is a form of defective colour vision in which three primary colours (red, green, and blue) are necessary to see any colour but the proportions of each primary are not the same as those required by a normal. Dichromatism is a form of colour vision deficiency in which all colours can be matched by a mixture of only two primary colours.

In *protanomaly*, a high proportion of red is needed when mixing red and green to match a yellow, whereas in *deuteranomaly* a high proportion of green is needed; the latter case being the most common type of congenital colour defect. *Tritanomaly* is where an abnormally high proportion of blue is needed when mixing blue and green to match a given blue–green stimulus. *Protanopia* is a condition in which only two hues are seen; below 495 nm all radiations appear bluish, whereas above it they all appear yellowish. Hence the colours confused will be reds, oranges, blue–greens, and greys. *Deuteranopia* is a condition in which red and green are confused; the longer wavelengths appear yellow and the shorter wavelengths appear blue. *Tritanopia* is a very rare condition in which blue and yellow are confused; the reds, the bluish greens, and greens are seen clearly.

Colour is commonly used to code information, and hence the correct identification of colours may be very important for efficient work. It is also used with hazard warnings and safety messages. For example, the contents of fire extinguishers, pipelines, electric cable, and micro-electronic components are all colour-coded. Colour-coding can also be used in sorting tasks and filing systems, as it can reduce search times and improve efficiency. Tasks involving the judgement of colour can be divided into four classes (Cole 1973):

1. *Comparative judgements of colour.* When precise matches of colour are made or subtle colour differences need to be appreciated, e.g. mixing dye stuffs to match a sample.

2. *Connotative recognition of colour.* When colour is used to code information, e.g. signal lights.

3. *Denotative colour recognition.* Where colour is used to identify an object. It is often used in filing systems or in sorting tasks.

4. *Aesthetic colour judgements.* Where colours are selected for their harmonious effects or evocative qualities, e.g. interior decorating, the advertising industry.

Guidelines have been given concerning the suitability of people with colour vision defects for certain occupations. Appendix A (p. 203) summarizes these guidelines (Voke 1980).

Depth perception

The visual system can effectively judge the distance of objects using both monocular and binocular cues, the latter being the most sensitive measure. A perception of depth can be achieved by a monocular subject from the following cues: geometric perspective, aerial perspective, interposition, distribution of light and shade, interpretation of size, and parallax. The binocular cues to depth are stereopsis (by utilizing the small angular disparity between the two eyes), and convergence.

Obviously, depth perception is not necessary for all tasks but stereopsis is of vital importance for jobs utilizing stereoscopic viewing instruments, e.g. aerial contour photography and binocular microscopy and for other jobs such as fork-lift truck operator, crane driver, and pilot. Hofstetter and Bertsch (1976) found that stereopsis does not decline between 8 and 46 years of age. However, beyond 46 it does appear to decline (Bell *et al.* 1972). More studies with larger numbers of subjects are needed to settle the relationship between age and stereopsis.

Depth perception can be affected by such factors as uncorrected refractive errors, uncompensated muscle balances, amblyopia, anisometropia, and squints. At low levels of illumination depth perception is of a very low order, which may be a problem for some occupations, e.g. photographers who need to cut photographic papers or pour chemical solutions in a dark room. In such circumstancese extra care needs to be taken to avoid accidents (Grundy, 1988).

Also of great importance for maximum visual comfort when performing a task is the stability of binocular vision, expecially for near tasks. Stress may be caused by an uncompensated excessive horizontal or vertical phoria. Heterophorias can be induced by prolonged periods of work. Some studies have reported an increase in esophoria after sustained fixation at near (Stenhouse-Stewart 1945; Ehlrich 1987). Stress may also be caused by deficiencies in the fusional reserves or due to a low near point of convergence when near tasks are being carried out.

The advantages of binocular vision over monocular vision are: (i) the presence of stereopsis; (ii) improved visual acuity; (iii) a lower absolute threshold; (iv) a closer near point of accommodation; (v) an enlarged field of peripheral vision; and (vi) slightly brighter perception of objects.

Visibility of tasks

The ability to perform a task safely, efficiently and comfortably depends upon its visibility, as well as on the visual capabilities of the employee, as outlined. Naturally, the better the visibility, the easier it is to perform the task, and the factors that influence the visibility of a task can be listed as follows:

(1) size of task;

(2) distance of task;

(3) illumination;

(4) contrast;

(5) colour;

(6) time available to view task;

(7) movement of the task;

(8) glare;

(9) atmospheric conditions.

How these factors affect visibility has been investigated by many researchers using different methods. One method is indirect: the influence of lighting, contrast, size of task, etc. upon job performance is assessed by measuring, for example, speed and accuracy. The simplest of the factors to adjust is the illumination, and therefore many studies have investigated its influence. The aim is to establish the range of lighting conditions that permits an improvement in job performance. With any study, either in a real environment or laboratory-simulated conditions, certain factors must be taken into account and controlled if possible, e.g. motivation, methods of payment of employees, and type of work (and therefore level of visual difficulty of the task). There are other problems that are encountered in studies in the real environment (Henderson and Marsden 1972):

1. It is difficult to define the contrast in a task by reflectances from the detail and background because it is rare for the surfaces to be perfectly matt.

2. The exposure time can be hard to control. The viewing time allowed for many tasks is not externally controlled.

3. The size of the task can be variable. It can be altered by the employee moving closer to the task and hence increasing the angular subtense at the eye.

One study in particular has influenced the lighting codes of Britain: Weston (1945) assessed the effects of illumination upon a self-paced scanning task. The observers viewed an array of 256 Landolt rings, the gaps of which were randomly arranged in one of eight directions and they were asked to cancel all the rings with a gap in a specific orientation. The total time taken and the number of errors made, along with the number of appropriate rings missed, were recorded. Allowing for the time required for physically cancelling the rings it was then possible to give a value of performance in terms of speed and accuracy. The test was repeated using different levels of illumination, different contrasts between the rings and their background and different ring sizes. The results are presented in Figure 1.6, which shows the mean performance for different contrast, size and illumination producing relative visual performance curves. Four main conclusions can be drawn from the results:

1. Increasing the illumination produces an increase in performance, but this follows the law of diminishing returns, i.e. smaller and smaller

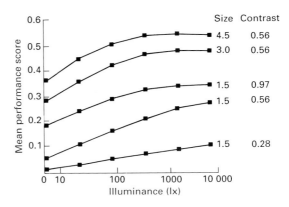

Fig. 1.6 Mean performance scores for Landolt ring charts (after Weston 1945).

changes in performance until no further improvement occurs and there may be a decrease in performance due to disability glare.

2. The point of the maximum performance is different for rings of different sizes and contrast. The smaller the size and the lower the contrast, the higher the level of illumination at which maximum performance occurs.

3. Larger improvements in performance can be achieved by changing the task size or contrast than by increasing the illumination.

4. Increasing the illumination does not make a visually difficult task, i.e. small size and poor contrast, reach the same level of performance as a visually easy task.

Although the findings above do, in principle, apply to all tasks, the relationship between illumination on the task and performance achieved will vary according to the type of task. In summary, the effect of illumination upon task performance will vary according to:

(1) the visual difficulty of the task;

(2) the extent to which the visual part of the task determines the overall performance.

The greater the visual difficulty, the greater the effect of the illuminance, whereas in a task such as audio typing, where there is only a small visual component, the effect of illuminance upon the overall task performance will be small.

To determine the optimum illumination levels for a task, the contrast and size need to be measured and, as mentioned, it is not easy to measure the contrast of a practical task. Weston therefore developed a simplified method, which avoided measuring the task contrast. He used 0.9 reflectance to give one contrast curve, which meant that only the size needed to be measured. This provided the basis for the illumination standards in the CIBS code (1984). These recommendations apply to tasks of normal contrast and reflectance. If, however, the contrast or reflectances are low, or if mistakes are made due to wrong perception and these are likely to be dangerous or costly, the recommended illumination should be increased.

Studies by Blackwell and Blackwell (1971) concerning the visibility of tasks have influenced the American codes for lighting. The initial experiments carried out investigated the threshold detection of static disc targets, and later experiments involved the detection of dynamic targets. The dynamically presented targets were believed to create conditions more similar to a practical task. More recent studies have investigated the effects of lighting upon the visual performance of a 20–30-year-old age group (Blackwell and Blackwell 1980).

Older individuals require more light than younger ones to perform a similar task. This is partly due to the fact that, with increasing age, senile miosis and lowered transmission of the ocular media (especially the crystalline lens) reduce the light reaching the retina and also increase the light scatter. There is a three-fold reduction in the amount of light reaching the retina of a 60-year-old compared to that of a 20-year-old (Weale 1961). The scattering of light means that glare becomes more of a problem with

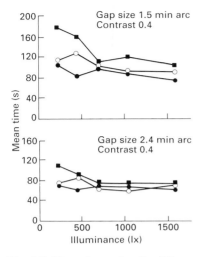

Fig. 1.7 Mean times taken for different age groups examining Landolt ring charts. ● 16–30 years; ■ 31–45 years; ◆ 46–50 years (reproduced by kind permission of P.R. Boyce and The Chartered Institute of Building Services 1973).

age, especially after the age of 40 (Wolf 1960; Reading 1968; Paulson Sjostand 1980). Further work has been carried out by Weston (1949), who investigated the effect of age upon visual performance at various lighting levels. The results showed a decrease in visual performance with age, but the performance of the older workers improved as the illumination was increased. A study by Boyce (1973) on a larger number of workers has also confirmed these findings for similar static tasks. The mean time taken by different age groups to read through Landolt C charts of different size, contrast, and illumination was measured. When the performance of older workers is compared with younger ones the difference between the groups diminishes as the illumination is increased (Fig. 1.7). While older workers generally gain more from an increase in illumination, it is unclear whether the same level of performance can be achieved by all ages by simply increasing the illumination. Boyce (1973) found no significant difference between the age groups at the highest illuminances used (up to 10 000 lx).

The effect of veiling reflections and the complexity of the task have a significant effect on job performance. Veiling reflections are due to light from a high luminance surface, such as a luminaire, being reflected from a specular surface, which is being viewed. These veiling reflections cause a reduction in performance due to the decreased contrast created on the task by the superimposed reflections.

The ability to discriminate colours is particularly influenced by age and illumination. It has been shown that with age there are more errors in hue discrimination in the blue–green and red regions (Verriest *et al.* 1962). Similar effects have been found by Boyce (1977), who also found that the older age group made more errors in sorting the hues in the FM 100 hue test and that the number of errors decreased with increasing illumination.

The time available to see the task is important; too short a time exposure will reduce the visibility, especially if the task is moving.

Atmospheric conditions in such industries as foundries and mining, where there may be dust, smoke, or steam will reduce visibility due to the absorption of light.

It is worthwhile mentioning that workers with poor visual acuity may also benefit from increased lighting levels (Silver *et al.* 1980; Julian 1984) and from more magnification to increase the retinal image size. As the majority of people with visual impairment are past the retirement age, the work that they undertake is mainly of a domestic nature. People with macular degeneration, a common cause of low visual acuity in the elderly, do benefit from an increase in illumination level (Sloan 1969; Sloan *et al.* 1973). The visual acuity was found to increase with an increase of luminance of the task up to 300 cd/m². A high level of illumination may also allow people to read continuous text without the aid of a magnifier, or with less magnification than normally required at lower levels of illumination. People with a loss of peripheral vision, commonly due to open-angle glaucoma, are more difficult to help. The problem that they experience is of orientation and location of objects. Of most benefit to these workers is the provision of good contrast between objects and the background. For example, door frames and door handles should be a different colour to the door itself. The edge of a step should also be highlighted, for example by a white strip on a dark step (Jay 1980). The use of different colours, sizes, and shapes may also be useful to distinguish different containers. Objects are also more easily detected if a plain rather than patterned background is used (Sicurella 1977).

To summarize, the illumination, size, and contrast of the critical detail of the task have a marked influence upon job performance. But other factors must not be forgotten, such as veiling reflections, complexity of the task, and motivation. Whilst lighting is one of the easiest factors to adjust to improve visibility, it must be remembered that a greater increase in visibility may be achieved by altering the contrast or the size of the task. Also, the idea that the higher the level of lighting the better the visibility is not always the case, as visibility may be reduced by disability glare.

Visibility meters

The principle of visibility meters is to reduce the visibility of a task to threshold and then relate the amount of reduction to a measure of visibility. Visibility meters can be used in several ways:

1. They can assess the relative visibility of a task and compare it to a standard condition.

2. Once the level of visibility is established, they can be used to assess how much illumination is required to make the task as visible as the standard.

3. The effects of illumination, contrast, colour, and polish of objects on the visibility can be assessed immediately.

Some meters reduce the visibility of the task to threshold by increasing the amount of veiling luminance and simultaneously decreasing the luinance from the task. This means that the overall luminance at the observer's eye does not change, nor does the state of adaptation of the eye (see Fig. 1.8). A variable beam splitter can be used to achieve this effect. The visibility metre designed by Eastman (1968) uses a glass plate with varying amounts of chromium alloy vapourized on it for this. The veiling luminance is provided by either the task background or a standard reflecting surface placed beside the task. Other meters use an internal light source to provide the veiling luminance.

Practical lighting installations do not generally produce completely diffuse illumination, and it is therefore necessary to have a measure of the extent to which lighting conditions differ from reference conditions. The contrast rendering factor (CRF) is a measure of the relative visibility under actual lighting conditions compared with the relative visibility under reference lighting conditions. (Reference lighting can be defined as that provided by an intergrating sphere where light is incident equally from all directions.) The CRF can be measured by viewing a task through a visibility meter. So the task is first viewed under the actual lighting conditions, and the visibility is reduced to threshold by increasing the veiling luminance. The relative visibilty of the target is equal to:

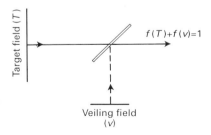

Fig. 1.8 Visibility meter. $f(T)$ fraction of total luminance from the target field reaching the observers eye; $f(v)$ fraction of total luminance from the veiling field reaching the observer's eye, $f(T) + f(v) = 1$. (After Eastman 1968.)

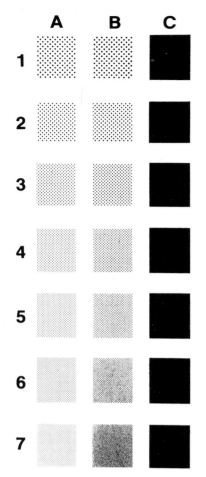

Fig. 1.9 Visibility indicator. Copyright J.W. Grundy (1989).

$$\frac{\text{Total luminance}}{\text{Luminance from target field}} \qquad (1.2)$$

The relative visibility of the same task is measured under reference lighting conditions with the same adaptation luminance at the person's eye. The CRF can then be calculated and will have a value between zero and one; the nearer to 1 the closer the actual conditions are to the reference conditions.

A simple, inexpensive, visibility indicator that can be used to determine whether lighting levels for near vision tasks are adequate, has been designed by Grundy (1989) (Fig. 1.9). It is a card with dots of decreasing size and three different contrast levels (high, medium, and low). It can be used to compare the visual performance under lighting conditions in an optometrist's practice to those at home or work. The visual capability is assessed by asking the person to look down each of the three columns of different contrast levels in turn, until the dots can no longer be seen. This should be carried out under the recommended lighting level with any near prescription required and in the same position and distance as the task to be assessed. If a light metre is not available to measure the illumination level, an approximate guide as to the level, which may be provided by a 60- and 100-watt bulb in a simple reflector such as an angle-poise, is given in Table 1.3 (Grundy 1989). A note is made on the card where the dots can no longer be seen and the test is then repeated by the person in the work or home situation. If the visibility is poorer at work or at home, it may be that the illumination level is inadequate and that an additional light source will improve the visibility.

Table 1.3 Approximate levels of illumination (lux) that can be expected from 100 W and 60 W pearl bulbs (reproduced by kind permission of J.W. Grundy and *Optometry Today* 1989)

	Distance (cm)							
	30	40	50	60	70	80	90	100
60 watt	900	500	320	225	165	125	100	80
100 watt	1800	1000	640	450	330	250	200	160

Summary

Many factors that influence visual performance, Figure 1.10 summarizes the major ones. These are factors inherent in both the observer and the task itself. For maximum visual performance, the task and the worker should be assessed so as to match the requirements of the task with the visual capabilities of the worker.

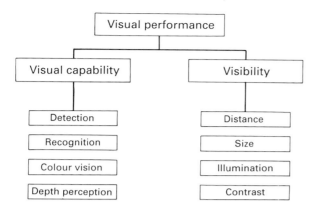

Fig. 1.10 Major factors that influence the visual performance.

References

Arundale, K. (1978). An investigation into the variation of human contrast sensitivity with age and ocular pathology. *Br. J. Ophthalmol.*, **62**, 213–15.

Axelrod, S. (1963). Cognitive tasks in several modalities. In *Processes of aging*, Vol. 1 (ed. R.H. Williams, C. Tibbits and W. Donahue), pp. 132–45. Atherton, New York.

Bell, B., Wolf, E., and Bernholz, D. (1972). Depth perception as a function of age. *Aging Hum. Dev.*, **3**, 77–81.

Bishop, H.P. and Crook, M.H. (1961). *Absolute identification of colour for targets presented against white and coloured backgrounds.* USAF WADC Report 60–611. In *Vision and its protection. A symposium on visual efficiency and eye protection at work*, (ed. E.C. Wigglesworth and B.L. Cole), (1973). Chapter 1. Australian Optometrical Publishing Company.

Blackwell, O.M. and Blackwell, H.R. (1971). Visual performance data for 156 normal observers of various ages. *J. Illum. Eng. Soc.*, **1**, 3–13.

Blackwell, H.R. and Blackwell, O.M. (1980). Population data for 140 normal 20–30 year olds for use in assessing some effects of lighting upon visual performance. *J. Illum. Eng. Soc.*, **9**, 158–74.

Botwinick, J. (1978). *Aging and behaviour*, (2nd edn). Springer, New York.

Boyce, P.R. (1973). Age, illuminance, visual performance and preference. *Ltg Res. Technol.*, **5**, 125–39.

Boyce, P.R. and Simons, R.H. (1977). Hue discrimination and light sources. *Ltg Res. Technol.*, **9**, 125–140.

Brozek, J. and Keys, A. (1945). Changes in flicker fusion frequency with age. *J. Consult. Psychol.*, **9**, 87–90.

Burg, A. (1966). Visual acuity as measured by dynamic and static tests. *J. Appl. Psychol.*, **6**, 460–6.

Burg, A. (1968). Lateral visual field as related to age and sex. *J. Appl. Psychol.*, **52**, 10–15.

CIBS Code for interior lighting (1984). 5th Edition. The Chartered Institution of Building Service Engineers, Lighting Division, London.

Cole, B.L. (1973). The handicap of abnormal vision. In Vision and its protection. A symposium on visual efficacy and eye protection at work (ed. E.C. Wigglesworth and B.L. Cole), pp. 37–43. Australian Optometrical Publishing Company, Sydney.

Davson, H. (1990). *Davson's Physiology of the eye*. (5th edn). Macmillan Press, London.

Domey, R.G. and McFarland, R.A. (1961). Dark adaptation as a function of age and individual prediction. *Am. J. Ophthal.*, **51**, 1262–8.

Drance, S.M., Berry, V., and Hughes, A. (1967). Studies on the effect of age on the central and peripheral isopters of the visual field in normal subjects. *Am. J. Ophthal.*, **63**, 1667–72.

Eastman, A.A. (1968). A new contrast threshold visibility meter. *J. Illum. Eng. Soc.*, **63**, 36–40.

Ehlrich, D.L. (1987). Near vision stress: vergence adaptation and accommodative fatigue. *Ophthal. Physiol. Optics*, **7**, 353–7.

Fergenson, P.E. and Suzansky, J.W. (1973). An investigation of dynamic and static visual acuity. *Perception*, **2**, 343–56.

Fletcher, R.J. (1961). *Ophthalmics in industry*, Chapter 5. Hatton Press, London.

Grey, R.H.B., Burns-Cox, C.J., and Hughes, A. (1989). Blind and partial sight registration in Avon. *Br. J. Ophthal.*, **73**, 88–94.

Grundy, J.W. (1981). Visual efficiency in industry. *Ophthal. Optician*, **21**, 548–52.

Grundy, J.W. (1987). A diagrammatic approach to occupational optometry and illumination. *Optom. Today*, Aug. 1st, 503–8.

Grundy, J.W. (1988). Prescribing and patient management: occupational and recreational considerations. In *Optometry*, (ed. K. Edwards and R. Llewellyn). Butterworths, London.

Grundy, J.W. (1989). A visibility indicator. *Optom. Today*, Nov. 20, 6–10.

Gunkel, R.D. and Gouras, P. (1963). Changes in scotopic visibility thresholds with age. *Arch. Ophthalmol.* **69**, 4–9.

Haas, A., Flammer, J., and Schneider, U. (1986). Influence of age on the visual fields of normal subjects. *Am. J. Ophthal.*, **101**, 199–203.

Hecht, S. (1934). Vision II. The nature of the photoreceptor process. In *A Handbook of general experimental psychology*, (ed. C. Murchinson). Clark University Press, Worcester, Mass.

Hills, B.L. (1975). *Some studies of movement perception, age and accidents*. Report SR137, Department of the Environment, TRRL, Crowthorne, Berkshire, UK.

Hofstetter, H.W. and Bertsch, J.D. (1976). Does stereopsis change with age?. *Am. J. Optom. Physiol. Optics.* **53**, 644–67.

Jay, P.A. (1980). Fundamentals. In *Light for low vision*, Proceedings of the Symposium held at University College, London on 4th April 1978, (ed. R. Greenhalgh), pp. 13–29. Partially Sighted Society, Doncaster, UK.

Julian, W.G. (1984). Variation in near visual acuity with illuminance for a group of 27 partially sighted people. *Ltg Res. Technol.*, **16**, 34–41.

Ludvigh, E. and Miller, J.W. (1958). Study of visual acuity during the ocular pursuit of moving test objects. 1. Introduction. *J. Opt. Soc. Am.*, **48**, 799–802.

McFarland, R., Domey, R.G., Warren, A.B., and Ward, D.C. (1960). Dark adaptation as a function of age. 1. A statistical analysis. *J. Gerontol.*, **15**, 149–54.

Millodot, M. and Millodot, S. (1989). Presbyopia correction and the accommodation in reserve. *Ophthal. Physiol. Optics.*, **9**, 126–32.

Paulson, L.E. and Sjostand, J. (1980). Contrast sensitivity in the presence of a glare light. *Invest. Ophthal. Vis. Sci.*, **19**, 401–6.

Reading, V.M. (1968). Disability glare and age. *Vision. Res.*, **8**, 207–14.

Riggs, L.A. (1965). Visual acuity. In *Vision and Visual perception*, (ed. C.H. Graham), pp. 321–49. Wiley, New York.

Robinson, D.A. (1968). The oculomotor control system: a review. Proc. I.E.E.E. **56**, 1032–49.

Sharpe, J.A. and Sylvester, T. (1978). Effect of aging on horizontal smooth pursuit. *Invest. Ophthal. Vis. Sci.*, **17**, 465–8.

Sicurella, V.J. (1977). Colour contrast as an aid for visually impaired persons. *Visual Impairment and Blindness*, **71**, 252.

Silver, J.H., Gould, E.S., Irvine, D., and Cullinan, T.R. (1980). Visual acuity at home and in eye clinics. *Ophthal. Optician*, **20**, 4.

Sloan, L.L. (1969). Variation of acuity with luminance in ocular diseases and anomalies. *Documenta. Ophth.*, **20**, 384.

Sloan, L.L., Habel, A., and Feiock, K. (1973). High illumination as an auxillary reading aid in diseases of the macula. *Am. J. Ophthal.*, **76**, 745–57.

Spooner, J., Sakala, S., and Bahol, R. (1980). Effect of aging on eye tracking. *Arch. Neurol.*, **37**, 575–6.

Stenhouse-Stewart, D.D. (1945). Some observations on a tendency to near point esophoria and possible contributory factors. *Br. J. Ophthal.*, **29**, 37–42.

Tiffin, J. (1945). Vision and industrial production. *Illum. Eng.*, **40**, 239.

Ungar, P. (1971). Sight at work. *Work Study*, **March**, 46–8.

Verriest, G., Vandevyvere, R., and Vanderdonck, R. (1962). Nouvelles reserches se rapportant a l'influence du sexe et de l'age sur la discrimination chromatique ainsi qu'a la signification practique des resultants du test 100 hue de Farnsworth–Munsell. *Res. D'Optique*, **41**, 499.

Voke, J. (1980). *Colour vision testing in specific industries and professions*. Keeler, London.

Weale, R.A. (1961). Retinal illumination and age. *Trans. Illum. Eng. Soc.*, **26**, 95–100.

Weale, R.A. (1963). *The ageing eye*. Lewis, London.

Weale, R.A. (1965). On the eye. In *Aging, behaviour and the nervous system*, (ed. A.T. Welford and J.E. Birren), pp. 307–25. C.C. Thomas, Springfield, Illinois.

Westheimer, G. (1987). Visual acuity. In *Adler's Physiology of the eye. Clinical application* (8th edn), Chapter 17, pp. 415–28. CV Mosby Co., St Louis.

Weston, H.C. (1945). *The relationship between illumination and visual performance*. Industrial Health Research Board Report No. 87. HMSO, London.

Weston, H.C. (1949). On age and illumination in relation to visual performance. *Trans. Illum. Eng. Soc.* (London) **16**, 281.

Weston, H.C. (1962). *Sight light and work* (2nd edn). Lewis, London.

Wolf, E. (1960) Glare and age. *Arch. Ophthalmol.*, **64**, 502–14.

Further reading

Boyce, P.R. (1981). *Human factors in lighting*. Applied Science Publishers, London.

Henderson, S.T. and Marsden, A.M. (ed.) (1972). *Lamps and Lighting*, (2nd edn). Edward Arnold, London.

Moses, R.A. and W.M. Hart (ed.) (1987). *Adler's physiology of the eye. Clinical application*, (8th edn). CV Mosby Co., St Louis.

Overington, I. (1976). *Vision and acquisition. Fundamentals of human visual performance, environmental influences and applications in instrumental optics*. Pentech Press, London.

Rosenbloom, A.A. and Morgan, M.W. (ed.) (1986). *Vision and aging. General and clinical perspectives*. Professional Press Books, New York.

Sekuler, R., Kline, D., and Dismukes, K. (ed.) (1982). *Aging and human visual function*. Alan Liss Inc., New York.

Weale, R.A. (1963). *The ageing eye*. Lewis, London.

2. Vision screening

The general purpose of any vision screening programme is to detect those people who have defective vision but who do not present with symptoms that result in them seeking attention. Every occupation has specific visual requirements that must be met to perform tasks efficiently, safely, and with comfort. Therefore the main aim of screening is to detect those people whose visual ability is below the standard required. Vision screening programmes are generally carried out either by government organizations, such as education authorities and the forces, or by employers. For instance, vision screening is commonly used to identify young children with defective vision, which can affect their progress at school.

There are a suprisingly high number of people with defective vision. The need for vision screening has been clearly demonstrated by the results of several surveys, which have shown that, on average, one-third of employees in industry have visual defects and are, therefore, presumed to be operating less efficiently (Rousell 1979; Grundy 1986). In fact, a study by Grundy (1984) found that 40.87 per cent of the employees whose task was to inspect piston rings for flaws were referred for full eye examination after a vision screening. The main reason for referral was found to be defective near vision. In general the employees were unaware of their visual deficiencies and had never considered that their vision might not have been adequate for the task. The prevalence of vision defects in school children increases with age and has been reported to be about 30 per cent at 14 years of age (Walters 1984). It would therefore appear from these studies that vision screening is indeed a worthwhile exercise.

Advantages to industry of vision screening

Bailey (1973) and Collins (1983) concur in their assessment of the advantages to industry of vision screening. These can be summarized as follows:

1. Selection of personnel. Visual ability can be used in the selection of new employees or the transfer of an employee to a task they can perform efficiently.

2. Identify employees with visual disabilities. These may be due to an uncorrected refractive error or ocular pathology. If the visual problems cannot be corrected then the employee can be transferred to a task they would be visually capable of performing efficiently.
3. Improved employee-employer relationship.
4. Improved visual efficiency can result in:
   (a) increased productivity;
   (b) fewer accidents and therefore reduced insurance costs;
   (c) reduced absenteeism as the task is less visually fatiguing.
5. Compensation claims can be settled more easily.

Given that an employer decides in favour of a vision screening programme, what steps need to be taken? First, visual standards for the various tasks must be established. This may be a relatively straightfoward procedure or, if the task is unique or highly complex, it may involve detailed analysis and assessment. Second, the method of screening must be selected, along with the appropriate tests. For advice on these matters a professional person, such as an optometrist, can be consulted.

Establishing occupational visual standards

There are two methods of determining the appropriate visual standard for a particular occupation, namely by the use of predetermined visual standards or by the establishment of the relationship between visual ability and job performance/competence.

Predetermined visual standards

Lists of standards of vision for various occupations may be found in the Association of Optometrists handbook and other optical diaries. Some standards are listed in the appendix of this book (see p. 210) and include such occupations as large goods vehicle and passenger carrying vehicle driving. Different tasks require different visual capabilities. For example, train drivers must be able to recognize certain colours whilst crane drivers need good depth perception. The standards listed can also be applied to occupations that are considered to have comparable visual requirements.

Relating visual ability to job competence

While it is quite simple to establish an employee's visual ability, relating this to their job competence is more complicated. There is no satisfactory method of grading job competence due to non-visual factors influencing the assessment. For example, it may be influenced by age, intelligence, attitude, motivation, manual dexterity, and motor reaction times. Bailey (1973) drew up a five-step programme for establishing the vision standard:

1. Choose a method for grading job competence.
2. Analyse the visual factors required for the task (see Visual Task Analysis, below).
3. Decide on criteria for visual competence, e.g. VA 6/9 or better, and stereopsis.

4. Screen the vision of two groups of employees who are judged to be:
   (a) job competent;
   (b) job incompetent.
   These two groups should be age-and sex-matched if possible.
5. Compare the grading of visual competence to job competence. If the appropriate vision standard has been chosen then the majority of the visually incompetent should fall into the job incompetent group.

Grading job competence can be done in a number of ways and Bailey (1973) suggests: (i) supervisor rating; (ii) quality and quantity of production; (iii) accident frequency; (iv) absenteeism; (v) employee turnover; (vi) wages (if on piece-rate).

Visual task analysis

Before the vision screening can be carried out there must be an analysis of the visual tasks involved in the occupation concerned. Analysing the visual factors required for the task is of crucial importance and ideally any analysis should be carried out at the place of work, e.g. factory or office. Factors such as distance and size of the critical detail of the task should be assessed, along with need for colour discrimination, depth perception, body, head and eye posture, field of vision, eye movements required, and the contrast and illumination of the task. From the subsequent analysis the important visual factors can be identified.

There are occasions when on-site analysis is not possible. A logical method for determining the visual factors required for a particular task has been proposed by Grundy (1987) and is designed to act as a simple reference guide for use by optometrists in a consulting room (Table 2.1).

From the knowledge of the distance and size of the critical detail of the task, the visual acuity necessary to discriminate the smallest detail can be determined. This can be calculated easily from a simple graphical method using a Nomogram, shown in Figure 2.1. For example, a task has a critical detail of 0.6 mm and it is viewed at 70 cm. When a straight line is drawn through these values it will intercept the right-hand scale to indicate that the corresponding visual angle is 3.0 min of arc and the minimum visual acuity required is 6/18. It is important to remember that the values given are a measure of the resolving power of the eye and higher standards are required for the task to be carried out for prolonged periods of time. It has been suggested that the visual acuity necessary for a demanding task should be approximately twice the minimum value (Grundy 1981). Therefore in the above case a visual acuity of 6/9 is advised. The employee can often move closer to the task, increasing the angular subtense at the eye, but this depends on the amount of accommodation and convergence available. The older presbyopic employee, who has a reduced amount of accommodation, may need an intermediate and a near prescription, depending on the distance of the task.

After analysis of the visual task allowing the important visual factors to be determined a standard can be set by either: (i) choosing a standard

Table 2.1 Occupational analysis (reproduced with kind permission of J.W. Grundy and *Optometry Today* 1987)

Name and general description of the task

Working distances	a. Far (beyond 200 cm) b. Intermediate (200–55 cm) c. Near (55–30 cm) d. Very near (Less than 30 cm)
Size of detail	a. Large (Angular size of critical detail over 10′) b. Medium (5′–10′) c. Small (3′–5′) d. Very small (2′–3′) e. Extremely small (1′–2′) f. Minute (less than 1′)
Main working positions	a. Sitting b. Standing c. Moving d. Mixture
Size of working areas (in which critical vision is required)	a. Large b. Medium c. Small
Head movements	a. Side to side b. Up and down c. Mixture
Direction of gaze	a. Ahead b. Up c. Down d. Side e. Mixture
Changes in direction of gaze	a. Frequent b. Occasional c. Seldom
Movement of the task	a. Stationary b. Slow movement c. Fast
Potential danger	a. High risk b. Medium risk c. Low risk
Special accuracy or care	a. Required b. Limited requirements c. Not required
Binocular vision and stereoscopic requirements	a. Required b. Not important c. Monocular vision adequate
Colour vision requirement	a. Good colour discrimination required b. Limited requirements acceptable c. Not required
Visual fields	a. Good field required b. Fair field acceptable c. Not important
Visibility (i.e. the relationship between the size of detail, working distances, contrast, and time available for viewing the task)	a. Good b. Fair c. Poor
Type of lighting in use, its adequacy and suitability	
Eye protection requirements	a. Required b. Not required
Hazard(s)	a. Basic b. Impact 2 c. Impact 1 d. Molten metal e. Dust f. Gas g. Chemicals h. Radiation i. Laser j. Other

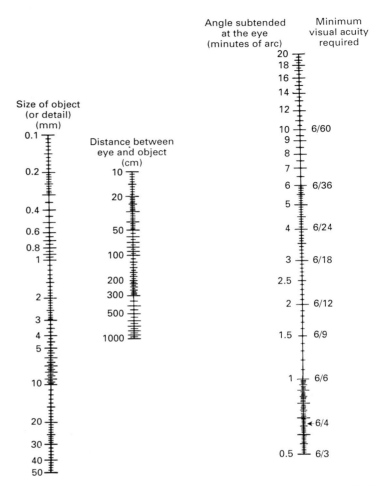

Fig. 2.1 Nomogram for finding the visual angle subtended by objects of which the size and distance are known (after Weston 1962).

believed to be necessary to work efficiently and safely, e.g. VA 6/12, distinguish principal colours. This can be tested by relating visual competence to job competence as described previously; or (ii) insisting on the normal level of visual capabilities for each factor chosen, e.g. VA 6/6, normal colour vision. This approach would exclude some who were capable of performing the task comfortably.

Methods of vision screening

Two techniques for screening vision may be used:

(1) modified clinical technique (MCT);

(2) instrument screeners.

Modified clinical technique

This method of screening is carried out by qualified personnel, e.g. optometrists, who assess the visual functions considered to be particularly important to job performance. The screening examination may therefore consist of any of the following (Bailey 1973; Collins 1983; Bennett and Rabbetts 1984):

1. *History and symptoms*. This is particularly useful as the history of a squint or amblyopic eye may be noted and this may reduce unneccessary referral. The presence of eyestrain when performing certain tasks can also be assessed.

2. *Visual acuity at any distance*. The measurement can be taken at the exact distance required, with the appropriate size of letters or task.

3. *External eye examination and ophthalmoscopy*. This allows detection of pathology of the eye that may otherwise go unnoticed. Ocular diseases do not always cause a reduction in vision that results in the person seeking medical attention.

4. *Retinoscopy*. This permits the precise degree of hyperopia or myopia to be assessed objectively. It will also indicate whether or not poor vision is due to the fact that spectacles are required.

5. *Amplitude of accommodation*. The result of this test will indicate whether the person can focus clearly and comfortably on a near task. Spectacles will generally be required, by the older presbyopic person, to see the task clearly.

6. *Binocular vision assessment*. This can include a cover test at the viewing distance required, motility, near point of convergence, and stereopsis. To avoid eyestrain, binocular vision needs to be stable and these tests will indicate whether the binocular functions are under stress for a particular task. The presence of a squint or phoria will be detected by the cover test.

7. *Visual field*. This can be assessed quite simply by a confrontation test, to determine whether there is any marked reduction, such as a homonymous hemianopia or quadrantic defects. The central visual field can be assessed using an Amsler Chart. When held at 30 cm, this chart covers the central 10 degrees of the field either side of fixation.

8. *Colour vision*. This can be assessed rapidly using tests such as the Ishihara Pseudo-isochromatic plates or Saturated D15. The Ishihara plates can be used to detect congenital colour vision defects and the Saturated D15 will detect acquired defects. However, if the task requires very fine discrimination of colours then a more thorough test, such as the FM100 Hue, may be used. For further details, regarding colour vision testing in industry and other professions see Voke (1980).

The MCT for vision screening has both advantages and disadvantages:

Advantages

1. Flexibility—tests can be selected depending on visual functions considered to be important for the task, and the tests can be performed at the appropriate distance.

2. Type and magnitude of refractive error can be assessed.
3. Ocular pathology may be detected.
4. Presence of a squint will be detected
5. Very few false referrals.

Disadvantages
1. Expensive method of screening due to the use of professional personnel, such as optometrists.
2. Time-consuming.
3. Shortage of professional people willing to participate in screening programmes.

Instrument vision screeners

There are many different instrument vision screeners available, but most are basically modified stereoscopes. The eye piece lenses are arranged so that their prismatic components simulate the viewing of a distant object and the near vision is simulated by either:

(1) moving the targets closer;
(2) decreasing the separation between the half stereograms;
(3) changing the lens power, i.e. introduce negative lenses.

The screeners usually have internal lighting and the targets are mounted either on a rotary drum or separately on cards, which are changed manually or by remote control. The types of tests commonly included in the instrument screeners are:

(1) visual acuity—distance and near (occasionally intermediate);
(2) heterophoria—horizontal and vertical at distance and near;
(3) stereopsis—distance and near;
(4) fusion;
(5) colour vision;
(6) fogging test;
(7) visual field;
(8) astigmatism.

Visual acuity
There are two methods used to assess the visual acuity, which is generally measured at distance and near:

(1) conventional letter charts, e.g. Illiterate Es;
(2) specially designed optotypes, i.e. checkerboard targets (Fig. 2.2).

Some of the optotypes used measure detectability and not the actual resolving power of the eye; this can be an advantage in some cases. For example, if the work involves the inspection of materials for holes or flaws, then a detectability test is a more suitable measurement of visual acuity.

Regardless of the type of target used for visual acuity assessment the results must be repeatable and provide valid measures. Results of several studies show that the distance visual acuity measures are repeatable,

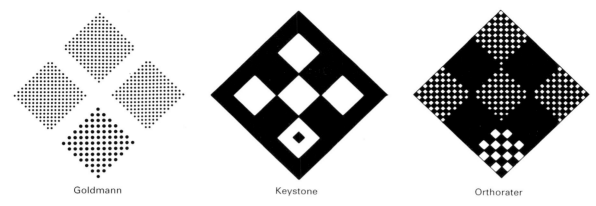

Goldmann   Keystone   Orthorater

Fig. 2.2 Optotypes (courtesy of D.B. Henson and Butterworth–Heinemann (Oxford) Ltd, 1983).

i.e. a high correlation is found between test and retest scores. Bailey and Cole (1968) investigated the validity of eight different vision screeners by comparing Snellen acuity measurements with those found from the screeners. They found that all but one of the screeners gave valid measures of the distance acuity.

Heterophoria

Many vision screeners include a test to measure the horizontal and vertical phorias. The test is generally based upon a dissociation technique, which can be used for distance and near measurements. Figure 2.3. shows an example of a horizontal and vertical phoria test. There is, unfortunately, a tendency for the distance phoria measured by the screeners to be relatively more esophoric than that found by conventional testing methods. This is due to the known proximity of the targets, which induces convergence, i.e. proximal convergence. The phoria test will also detect the presence of suppression as only one target will be seen, e.g. the arrow and not the letters.

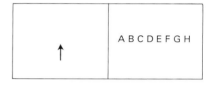

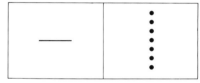

Fig. 2.3 Horizontal and vertical phoria test targets.

Stereopsis

Most of the instruments include a test of stereopsis, in which one of a series of targets presented to each eye is seen with a small retinal disparity. The observer reports which target appears to stand out and, with a series of such tests, each with a different size disparity, the stereo-acuity can be measured. Failure of the stereopsis test may be due to suppression or an uncorrected refractive error, or due to the artificially simulated viewing conditions. Therefore it cannot automatically be assumed that the observer has no, or poor, stereopsis if they fail the test. The person should be referred for further investigation when alternative tests can be used.

Fusion

Some instruments include a fusion test to assess the binocularity of the observer. This test presents similar targets to each eye but each has a control, i.e. one part of the target is only seen by the right eye and one part of the target is only seen by the left eye. For example, the Rodenstock screeners present a circle to each eye with a vertical line seen by one eye above the circle and a vertical line seen below the circle by the other. If the observer has fusion, one circle will be seen with a vertical line above and below the circle. If the observer has double vision two circles will be seen. The fusion test will also detect suppression, as only one target will be seen.

Colour vision

A series of isochromatic plates are included in most of the vision screeners to assess whether the observer has normal or defective colour vision. Unfortunately, due to the small number of plates used, the difficulty in accurate printing of the plates and the fact that tungsten lighting is often used instead of natural daylight, the sensitivity of the tests is low. It would seem more sensible to screen those who require colour vision separately, using the full set of isochromatic plates (Henson 1983). Some screeners test colour vision by the correct naming of colours.

Rodenstock vision screeners have a different test to screen for red and green colour vision defects. The test disc includes six bipartite test fields, i.e. each test field is divided into an upper and lower half. The observer has to state if the upper and lower test fields appear the same colour or different colours.

Fogging tests

These tests are used to detect hyperopic observers. Positive lenses are incorporated, which will blur or fog the target viewed by an emmetrope, e.g. + 1.50 D (Rodenstock R11, R12), + 1.75 D (VS-11 Vision Screener), or + 2.00 D (Mavis). A hyperope will find that the target is clear or see it more clearly than an emmetrope, depending upon the magnitude of the refractive error and object distance.

Visual field

The extent of the horizontal visual field is assessed by either of two methods:

1. *A perimeter attachment.* This is manually rotated about a point located on top of the screener (e.g. Rodenstock Screeners). The target is brought from behind the observer's head while they fixates a central point and the extent of peripheral vision is indicated on a dial.

2. *An electronic perimeter.* This has light-emitting diodes (LEDs) inset in a horizontal arc, either within the instrument (e.g. Keystone VS-II Vision screener) or in a separate attachment that can be placed on top of the instrument (e.g. Visiotest). The LEDs are illuminated by a push-button control and their positions usually extend from 85 degrees temporally to 45 degrees nasally. Figure 2.4 shows the compact Keystone VS-II Vision screener with the remote control unit. This operates the LEDs, which are positioned between the eye pieces and recessed in the temple areas of the head rest.

The Ergovision screener provides a more extensive test of the visual field. It presents each eye with ten luminous dots; four points in the central area, four points for the peripheral area and two points for the extent of the horizontal field.

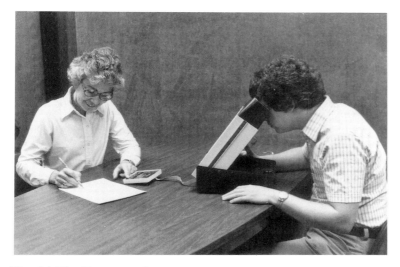

Fig. 2.4 The Keystone VS-II Vision Screener (courtesy of Warwick Evans Optical Co. Ltd).

Astigmatism

Only a few screeners include a test for astigmatism (e.g. Topcon screenoscope). These tests consist of:

1. A fan of lines with the observer having to state whether any appear blurred or if they are all clear.
2. The number of clear lines seen on the fan may be counted.

Two additional tests, very important for drivers, are featured in the Keystone Driver Vision Screener Model 2: (i) distance visual acuity; and (ii) stereopsis measurement under low illumination.

The Keystone and Rodenstock instruments offer a wide range of tests and are used by many organisations. The Ergovision screener incorporates many new tests as well as the conventional ones (Fig. 2.5). New tests have been included to gather data on such factors as dynamic visual acuity, variable contrast acuity, visual fatigue and dazzle recovery time. The instrument uses a voice synthesizer to carry out the standard tests and the results are printed out at the end of the programme. All the tests can also be carried out at three different lighting levels: 15, 150, 300 candelas/m^2. It is intended not as a diagnostic test but for studying vision in the working conditions. The wide range of tests should allow those visual examinations that are thought to be more closely matched to those of the task.

The Binoptometer is a vision screener which apparently overcomes the problem of proximal convergence. The tests are presented in free space, e.g. are seen against a distant wall and, hence, it eliminates proximal effects. This screener is currently available in Europe and is produced by Oculus. Also tests can be carried out at any distance varying from infinity to 0.3 m due to the optical design which is similar to a Badal Optometer.

A summary of some of the tests included in the currently available vision screeners is given in Table 2.2. For precise details see the manufacturers data. Lists of suppliers are included in Appendix B.

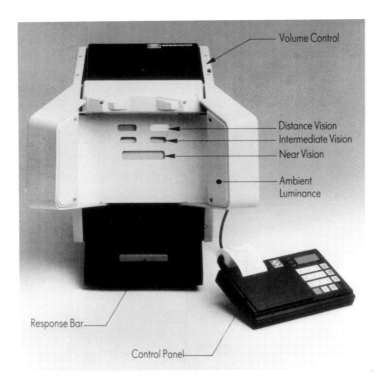

Fig. 2.5 The Ergovision Vision Screener (courtesy of Essilor Ltd).

Advantages of instrument vision screeners, Bailey (1973):
  (1) operated by lay technicians;
  (2) rapid screening;
  (3) always available for use;
  (4) low maintenance costs;
  (5) cheap method of screening.

Disadvantages of instrument vision screeners

  1. Lack of flexibility of tests and testing distance, especially for those screeners where the targets are on a rotary drum.
  2. Does not detect ocular pathology unless inferred by a reduction of visual acuity.
  3. Cannot detect squints.
  4. Awareness of the actual target distance may induce proximal accommodation and convergence, even when distance viewing conditions are simulated. This can effect the visual acuity measurement and induce a relative esophoria at distance.
  5. There can be unnecessary referral by a lay operator of people with amblyopia or a squint.

Choice of vision screening method

The ideal screening programme should:

Table 2.2 Summary of some of the currently available vision screeners

Screener Tests	Rodenstock			Keystone		Essilor		Optec 2000	Titmus II Vision Tester	Topcon Screenoscope SS-3	Oculus Binoptometer
	R10	R11	R12	VS II VS	Driver DVS II	Visiotest	Ergovision				
Acuity type	Checkerboard, Illiterate E, Numbers, Landolt C	Checkerboard, Illiterate E, Numbers, Pictures	Checkerboard, Illiterate E, Numbers, Landolt C	Numbers, Illiterate E	Numbers + low illumination	Letters Numbers	Letters Numbers	Checkerboard, Illiterate E, Landolt C	Landolt C	Illiterate E Landolt C	Landolt C
Phoria (H&V, D&N)	Yes	Yes	Yes	Yes	Yes at distance	Yes	Yes	Yes	Yes	Yes	Yes
Fusion	Yes	Yes	Yes	Yes	No	No	Yes	Yes	No	No	Yes
Stereopsis	Yes	Yes	Yes	Yes	Yes + low illumination	Yes	Yes	Yes	Yes	Yes	Yes
Colour vision	Yes	Yes	Yes	Yes	Yes	Yes	Yes	Yes	Yes	No	Yes
Fogging lens	No	Yes	Yes	Yes	No	Yes	Yes	Yes	No	Yes	No
Visual field	Yes	Yes	Yes	Yes	Yes	Yes	Yes	Yes	Yes	No	No
Astigmatism	No	No	No	No	No	Yes	Yes	No	No	Yes	No
Target change	Manual	Manual	Manual	Remote control	Remote control	Manual	Automatic or remote control	Manual	Remote control	Manual	Manual
Test distances	Distance only for drivers	Distance and 40 cm	Distance, 55 cm and 33 cm	6 m, 66 cm and 37 cm	6 m	5 m and 33 cm	5 m, 66 cm and 33 cm	6 m and 35 cm 76–50 cm with five lens sets	6 m and 37 cm 1 m to 50 cm with five lens sets	5 m and 30 cm Lenses for intermediate	Infinity to 30 cm
Comments	For drivers. Some test discs are interchangable between screeners, e.g. adult, industrial & driver discs	For children	For industry, VDU	VDU test Head position sensor	For drivers	VDU lens kit for 50 cm tests	Extra tests, e.g. visual fatigue, glare recovery, dynamic VA. Three light levels	Slide sets for industry, medical, international use. Head position sensor	Low light level. Head position sensor. Job standard manual	Job standard manual	VDU and driver test discs

(1) maximize screening success, i.e. correct referral and non-referral;

(2) minimize screening errors, i.e. low over and under referral rate. In other words the test needs good sensitivity and specificity.

The use of visual acuity measures alone as a method of screening children is not sensitive enough, especially when compared to the modified clinical technique (MCT) or use of instrument screeners (Hatcher 1976; Swarbrick 1979; Worrall 1981; Cohen *et al.* 1983). When the MCT was compared to the use of instrument screeners or a battery of vision tests, it was found to be the most sensitive, with the lowest under- and over-referral rate (Peters *et al.* 1959; Wick *et al.* 1976; Wong 1978; Cole and Robbins 1981; Worrall 1981). Therefore, when screening children, it appears that the MCT, although not infallible, is preferable, as it is less likely to over- or under-refer. Instrument screeners are widely used for vision screening of adults, and are often the method of choice used in industry and by government organizations. However, it must be remembered that whichever technique is used, it is only a screening test, and not a substitute for a full ophthalmic examination.

References

Association of Optometrists Members Handbook. Association of Optometrists, Bridge House, 233–4, Blackfriars Road, London, SE1 8NW.

Bailey, I.L. (1973). Vision screening in industry: objective and methods. *Aust. J. Optom.*, **56**, 70–85.

Bailey, I.L. and Cole, B.L. (1968). *Methods and instruments for screening distance and near acuity.* Victorian College of Optometry, University of Melbourne, Australia.

Bennett, A.G. and Rabbetts, R.B. (1984). *Vision screening, new subjective refractors and techniques. Clinical visual optics.* Butterworths, London.

Cohen, A.H., Lieberman, S., Stolzberg. M., and Ritty, J.M. (1983). The NYSOA vision screening battery—a total approach. *J. Am. Optom. Assoc.*, **54**, 975–84.

Cole, B.L. and Robbins, H.G. (1981). The problems of screening children's vision. *Aust. J. Optom.*, **64**, 193–6.

Collins, M. (1983). *Occupational public health optometry*, pp. 1–8. Department of Optometry, Queensland Institute of Technology, Brisbane, Queensland.

Grundy, J.W. (1981). Visual efficiency in industry. *Ophthal. Opt.*, **Aug 15**, 548–52.

Grundy, J.W. (1984). When your car could break down through a visual defect. *Ophthal. Opt.*, **Feb 4**, 77–80.

Grundy, J.W. (1986). A simple method of occupational vision requirements. *Optom. Today*, **Oct 11**, 684–8.

Grundy, J.W. (1987). A diagrammatic approach to occupational optometry and illumination. *Optom. Today*, **Aug 1**, 503–8.

Hatcher, M.J. (1976). A kindergarten vision screening service. *Aust. J. Optom.*, **59**, 198–201.

Henson, D.B. (1983). *Optometric instrumentation*, pp. 231–7. Butterworth–Heinemann Ltd, London.

Peters, H.B., Blum, H.L., Bettman, J.W., Johnson, F., and Fellows, V. (1959). The Orinda vision study. *Am. J. Optom. A.A.A.O.*, **36**, 455–69.

Rousell, D. (1979). *Eye protection.* Royal Society for the Prevention of Accidents Publication No. IS126. RoSPA, Birmingham.

Sasieni, L.S. (1979). A guide to vision screening instruments. *The Optician*, **Sept. 14**, 11–21.

Swarbrick, H.A. (1979). Vision screening in New Zealand schools. *Aust. J. Optom.*, **62**, 374–82.

Voke, J. (1980). *Colour vision testing in specific industries and professions.* Keeler Ltd, London.

Walters, J. (1984). Portsea modified clinical technique: evaluation of an expanded optometric vision screening protocol for children. *Aust. J. Optom.*, **67**, 212–20.

Weston, H.C. (1962). *Sight, light and work*, (2nd edn). Lewis, London.

Wick, B., O'Neal, M., and Ricker, P. (1976). Comparison of vision screening by lay and professional personnel. *Am. J. Optom. Physiol. Optics.*, **53**, 474–8.

Wong, S.G. (1978). Comparison of vision screening performed by optometrists and nurses. *Am. J. Optom. Physiol. Optics.*, **55**, 384–9.

Worrall, R.S. (1981). The Biopter vision test: use in school screening program. *Optom. Monthly*, **72**, 10–13.

3. Incidence of ocular injuries and their prevention

Incidence of ocular injuries

Recent studies show that there is still an unacceptably large number of eye injuries occuring in the UK (Canavan *et al.* 1980; Chiapella and Rosenthal 1985; Wykes 1988; MacEwen 1989). In the USA there is also concern about the large number of eye injuries, and the resultant effect on vision. One study, by the National Society for the Prevention of Blindness (1980) states that there are approximately 1 100 000 people in the USA with some type of visual impairment as a result of an eye injury. This may vary from only a slight reduction in visual acuity to total blindness, and in the latter case approximately 75 per cent of the patients are monocularly blind. Sadly, it also appears that the majority of these injuries could have been prevented; the NSPB estimated that 90 per cent of such injuries are preventable (National Society for the Prevention of Blindness 1984).

While in the past eye injuries have been associated with industrial occupations, there are now an increasing number due to sports and leisure activities. Obviously the number of eye injuries caused by industrial accidents will vary according to the level of industrialization in the area concerned. For example, a study in a heavily industrialized area (Wolverhampton, UK; Lambah 1968) reported that 73.8 per cent of all eye injuries over a ten-year period occurred in industry, compared to only 15.4 per cent reported in less industrialized Northern Ireland for a similar period (Canavan *et al.* 1980).

Canavan *et al.* (1980) carried out a survey into the cause and resultant type of ocular injury from 1967 to 1976. The causes of the ocular injuries of people admitted to the Royal Victoria Hospital, Belfast, were listed in order of decreasing frequency as follows:

(1) children at play and sport   33.8 per cent;
(2) road traffic accidents   19.3 per cent;

(3) industrial accident   15.4 per cent;

(4) civil disturbance   9.1 per cent;

(5) home accident   6.8 per cent;

(6) assault   6.8 per cent;

(7) adult sport   4.8 per cent;

(8) farm accident   4.0 per cent.

Of the 2032 patients admitted, 1707 were male and 325 female. Men younger than 36 years of age were subject to the highest percentage of injuries (77.4 per cent). Similar findings have been reported in other surveys (Chiapella and Rosenthal 1985; Wykes 1988; MacEwen 1989).

The survey also recorded the type of ocular injury:

(1) blunt injury   49.2 per cent;

(2) perforating injury   48.0 per cent;

(3) intra-ocular foreign body 8.4 per cent.

Normal visual acuity was regained in 41.2 per cent of known cases, but many resulted in severe loss of vision. Perforation of the eye accounted for the majority of cases with severe loss of vision. A common cause of perforating eye injuries used to be road traffic accidents, in which the head impacted upon the jagged edges of the shattered windscreen. However, since the introduction of compulsory wearing of seat belts in the UK in January 1983, there has been a significant decrease in this type of injury. Hall *et al.* (1985) found a 73 per cent reduction in such injuries; Cole *et al.* (1987), Johnson and Armstrong (1986), and Wykes (1988) have noted similar reductions.

Another large UK study (Chiapella and Rosenthal 1985) examined the clinical records of 6576 patients admitted to the eye casualty department at the Leicester Royal Infirmary during a one-year period. While, again, the majority of patients were men in the 20–40-year age group, the main cause of eye injuries was foreign bodies. Table 3.1 shows the main occupations of the patients in whom the injuries occurred. Press and machine tool operators were the most likely to suffer injury (32 per cent) However, is important to remember that most of the occupations listed are covered by the Protection of Eyes Regulations 1974, and that eye protection should have prevented injury! The study suggests that eye protection was either inappropriate or was not being used correctly by the workers.

Relatively few industrial processes do not present an ocular hazard of some type. Despite the fact that legislation demands eye protection during hazardous tasks, many ocular injuries still occur. The exact number of these injuries is difficult to ascertain because there is no general concensus for collecting data. Injuries are often not reported unless they result in a loss of time from work. In 1985, a total of 6982 major injuries were reported to Her Majesty's Factory Inspectorate which had occurred to employees in the manufacturing and construction industries (Health and Safety Executive 1988). Of the injuries, 269 (3.8%) were of an ocular nature. While the majority of the ocular injuries were superficial, there were significant numbers of perforating and contusion injuries.

Table 3.1 Occupations of the patients when the ocular injury occurred (reproduced by kind permission of A.P. Chiapelli and A.R. Rosenthal and the *British Journal of Ophthalmology* 1985)

Occupation	No. of cases				
	All injuries	Burn	Contusion	Foreign body	Corneal abrasion
Press or machine tool operators	494	13	13	425	64
Motor vehicle or aircraft mechanic	147	10	7	111	18
Metal worker	145	7	4	111	27
Construction	131	16	6	82	37
Sheet metal worker	124	3	3	108	12
Electrician	104	5	3	77	24
General labourer	120	6	5	79	34
Welder	97	9	3	72	18
Bus, coach or lorry driver	76	4	5	46	23
Others in processing	51	4	1	23	8
Painter and decorator	44	7	1	23	17

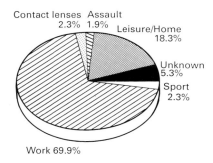

Fig. 3.1 Causes of ocular injuries (reproduced by kind permission of C.J. MacEwen and *The British Journal of Ophthalmology*, 1989).

Sadly, the incidence of industrial eye injuries does not appear to be reducing. A recent study by MacEwen (1989) found that 70 per cent of all eye injuries presenting over a 1-year period at the Glasgow Eye Infirmary and the Western Infirmary casualty departments had occurred at work. A total of 5671 patients were seen from May 1987 to April 1988. The distribution of the various causes of injury are shown in Figure 3.1. The most common occupation at the time of injury was grinding/buffing, and 83 per cent of all those injured were not wearing the required eye protection. Interestingly, whilst most injuries occurred at work, the majority of the serious injuries in this study were due to sporting and leisure activities.

Sport

The number of ocular injuries sustained during sport and leisure activities is on the increase. In the USA in 1983, there were an estimated 39 000 sport-related eye injuries. Not suprisingly there is a higher incidence of injury amongst the more hazardous sports, with baseball accounting for the greatest number (US, CSPC 1983). Hockey used to be a leading cause of eye injuries, but the numbers have decreased since the introduction of the mandatory use of protective face masks (Vinger 1980).

Racket sports are also responsible for many ocular injuries; this is not suprising, given the speed of the ball. A squash ball may reach speeds of 225 km/h (140 mph), a racket ball and tennis ball 177 km/h (110 mph), and a shuttle cock 233 km/h (145 mph). There is also the risk of the player being hit by the opponent's racket. Twenty-five per cent of injuries

Table 3.2 Distribution of ocular injuries resulting from sports seen at the Sussex Eye Hospital (reproduced by kind permission of P.T.S. Gregorg and the *British Journal of Ophthalmology* 1986)

Sport	Total accidents	Hospital admissions	Male	Female
Squash	24	3	18	6
Soccer	19	7	19	0
Badminton	16	4	6	10
Tennis	11	1	9	2
Rugby	6	0	6	0
Cricket	5	0	4	1
Basketball	3	0	1	2
Hockey	3	0	2	1
Golf	2	1	2	0
Marbles	1	1	1	0
Karate	1	0	1	0
Lacrosse	1	0	0	1
Total	92	17	69	23

received from racket sports are serious, and may result in permanent loss of vision. Racket sports have become the most common cause of eye injuries amongst women in the 20–50-year age group (Mills 1985).

Squash became very popular in Australia in the 1970s, which was reflected by the incidence of injuries; an amazing 32 per cent of all eye injuries admitted to the Royal Adelaide Hospital were received playing squash in the 30 months prior to November 1975 (Moore and Worthley 1977). The very high potential for ocular injury in squash is due not only to the fact that the squash ball can be travelling at very high speed, but also because it is small enough to fit into the orbit.

In the UK, a study by Gregory (1986) examined the distribution of sports of related eye injuries (Table 3.2). Squash is the most common source, with soccer, badminton, and tennis following closely behind. The majority of the injuries were to men, and 20 per cent of all patients were admitted to hospital. Cole *et al.* (1987) found that squash was the sport most often associated with perforating injuries, and in every case the injury was the result of wearing glass rather than plastic lenses.

Jones (1988) has reported that sport is becoming an increasingly important cause of severe eye injuries in the UK. In his year-long study of severe eye injuries admitted to the Manchester Royal Eye Infirmary, he found that racket sports accounted for half of the injuries (Fig 3.2). He also found that none of the patients had been wearing eye protection, and that they had no idea how to obtain it. Serious eye injuries to badminton

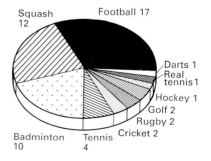

Fig. 3.2 Number of sports related eye injuries (reproduced by kind permission of N.P. Jones and *Eye* 1988).

players have also been reported by Kelly (1987), with damage being due to penetrating injuries from shattered glass spectacle lenses.

Unfortunately, there are cases where sportsmen have sight-threatening injuries of which they are unaware. A survey of 74 asymptomatic boxers showed that 58 per cent had a variety of ocular injuries, including traumatic cataracts and retinal tears (Giovinazzo et al. 1987). It is difficult to provide eye protection for boxers, but the report concluded that a more rigorous control of the sport is required, including regular eye examinations. The introduction of a thumbless boxing glove would help to reduce some of the injuries.

There can be no doubt about the necessity for eye protection in sport and the optometrist must be responsible for educating sportsmen and women about the potential hazards of their sport and the need for eye protection. This advice should be given to patients attending an optometric practice. The success of eye protectors in reducing ocular injuries has been demonstrated by the reduction in injuries to hockey players in the USA, as detailed by Vinger (1980). Eye protectors for racket sports have been developed in the USA and Canada and, apparently, no serious eye injury has been reported by a racket ball or squash player wearing the approved eye protectors (Easterbrook, 1988). Researchers have noted that open eye guards should not be used as the ball changes its shape in motion and flattens, so that it can make eye contact through the eye guard. In addition, spectacle frames with hinges that open beyond 90 degrees are not sufficiently rigid to prevent the frame from hitting the eye if it is struck by a racket or ball (Easterbrook 1981; Vinger 1985).

Children and domestic accidents

Many severe ocular injuries occur to children at play and in the home; such accidents are the major cause of blindness in the first two decades of life (Freeman 1979). A study by MacEwen (1989) found that a disproportionate number of serious eye injuries occurred to children.

La Roche et al. (1988) conducted an investigation into severe eye injuries in children. They found that young boys with perforating eye injuries accounted for the majority of cases involving severe loss of vision. Not surprisingly, the major cause of injury was due to objects being thrown, e.g. rocks, stones, snowballs, etc. BB gun pellets caused permanent loss of vision in almost half the cases seen (BB guns are a type of air gun that fire ball-bearings). The report concluded that adult supervision could have prevented most cases of permanent visual loss. The authors also suggested that legislation restricting the use of BB guns should be passed and that toy safety standards should be tightened. A programme of adult and child eye safety education should also be developed, and should include warnings of potentially hazardous toys, etc.

A similarly worrying report about eye injuries caused to children by guns was presented by Moore et al. (1987), who found that 70 per cent of ocular injuries caused by airguns occurred to the under 17-years age group. This emphasizes the need for parental control and education about the potential danger.

During the past ten years, hundreds of thousands of Americans have incurred eye injuries at home because they did not take safety precautions with potentially dangerous products (Randall 1985). Some of the household products cited in many eye injury reports include oven cleaners, glue, disinfectants, nylon cord grass trimmers, chain saws, hair sprays, paints, insecticides, and cleaning agents (e.g. ammonia, bleach). There are numerous potentially hazardous products in every home. Lawn mowers are resposible for a staggering number of injuries. John *et al.* (1988) found that, over a ten-year period from 1977–87, they were responsible for 70 000 injuries every year, and that 5 per cent of these involved the eyes.

Prevention of injuries

Role of optometrist/medical professions

In the USA a national Eye Trauma System has been formed to combat the problem of eye injuries in general (Parver 1988). This is composed of regional trauma centres with eye specialists always available to deal with severe ocular injuries. Data is also being collected to: (i) increase the knowledge of ocular trauma so that treatment techniques can be improved; and (ii) understand the mechanisms and circumstances that result in ocular injury so that effective protection can be provided.

The optometrist has an important role to play in the prevention of eye injuries. In practice, a thorough history of patients should be taken and a detailed analysis of the visual requirements made. What are the patients' hobbies? do they play sports? do they enjoy gardening? do they carry out DIY? do they ride a motorcycle or bicycle? what is their occupation and does this involve potential ocular hazards? From this information potential ocular hazards can be discussed, along with the need for eye protection where necessary (Woods 1988). The need for protective lenses for the patient with an amblyopic eye should not be forgotten.

The optometrist may also help reduce the number of injuries in industry by setting up Eye Protection Programmes. The success of such programmes has been demonstrated by the Norfolk and Western Company in the USA, which was unhappy with the number of injuries occuring to their employees and investigated the causes (Gross 1982). The accidents appeared to be due to the lack of mandatory eye safety programmes, unwillingness to wear eye protection, and the unfortunate assumption by both the management and employees that certain jobs were not potentially hazardous. After the introduction of an eye protection programme for employees in the mechanical and engineering departments in 1980, there was a 78.4 per cent reduction in eye injuries over the next three years.

Perception of Risk

It is well known that there is widespread wearer resistance to using eye protectors in hazardous industries (Farmer 1982). This was clearly shown in the survey by MacEwen (1989), who found that, in 85 per cent per cent of injuries that occurred at work, eye protection was not being worn when it should have been. There is concern that people do not take the available measures to protect their health in general and that health messages frequently do not achieve the desired effect. Various theories have been proposed to explain this attitude of indifference to health hazards. The Health Belief Model was put foward by Rosenstock *et al.* (1959), suggesting that a person's behaviour depended on various factors such as: the degree of perceived risk, the perceived benefits of taking preventative measures, and the perceived barriers, e.g. inconvenience. A more recent model, the dual Process Model, emphasizes the role of a person's experience based on past personal knowledge and the information from friends, colleagues, the media, and their doctor (Levanthal *et al.* 1983). Hence it concentrates on how an individual's, 'perceptions' relevant to the Health Belief Model are formed. If the risk of receiving an eye injury is perceived as high, a person is more likely to wear an eye protector. It is suggested that an individual learns to appreciate risks through experiencing either an injury to themselves or a friend (Powell *et al.* 1971). Hence a worker who has not had such a past experience will generally perceive the risk as being moderate. However, this is not always the case. In one study, a decreased perception of risk was found in workers who had survived, or who had seen others survive, eye injuries (Gervais 1989). This study investigated the relationship between past experience of eye injuries in chemical industry workers and their attitude towards the use of safety spectacles. The publicizing of eye injuries as a warning might have a negative effect, as in some cases the worker will inform colleagues that 'it wasn't actually so bad'. In other cases the effect of 'near misses', was useful, as there was a clear association between having eye sight saved by eye protection and perceived risk. Caution must therefore be exercized when publicizing eye injuries as a warning to workers. From the study, the following recommendations to promote eye safety were made.

1. Educational efforts should be directed at the younger employees, as they are less convinced about the risk they run when not wearing eye protection. Note that they often do not have the added benefit of improved vision through the use of prescription safety spectacles.

2. The publicizing of eye injuries must be considered carefully.

3. It may be beneficial to counsel workers after an eye injury to determine the perception of risk of their occupation. If their perception of risk is low, then efforts can be made to instruct them as to the hazards so that, hopefully, they will be more inclined to wear their eye protection.

4. Reasons for not wearing eye protection should be determined.

5. The possibility of compulsory wear should not be overlooked, but it should not be enforced in a heavy-handed manner.

Eye protection programme

In the past the safety of the employee was normally considered to be the employee's responsibility, and little liability was placed upon the employer. However, in more recent years the trend has been reversed and the employer is primarily responsible for the safety of the employees. This has led to claims for compensation, fines, and obligations to provide financial support during absence from work, as well as the cost of lost production. It has therefore became worthwhile for employers to invest in accident prevention programmes. The main aim of an eye protection programme is to identify potential ocular hazards and then to eliminate or control them. This will not only fulfil legal obligations but will also have economic advantages (Collins 1983). A reduction in eye injuries will result in a reduction of insurance and medical expenses. There will be a reduction in lost production, work replacement, and retraining costs for those who, due to injury, cannot continue in their previous job. An improvement in the employee/employer relationship may also result from the instigation of an eye protection programme. The prevention of the devastating effects that visual impairment causes to both the employee and their family, should not be forgotten.

Naturally, the expenses incurred in developing such a programme will have to be evaluated. These will include the fees for a consultant to carry out the initial survey and the cost of implementation. This may involve modifying manufacturing processes to either eliminate or control the hazards; this may be expensive. There is the cost of providing and maintaining eye protection for employees and, finally, there is the cost of employee education concerning ocular hazards of their jobs and use of eye protectors where necessary (Gross 1982; Nakagawara 1988).

The eye protection programme may contain the following parts (Lathey 1973; Taylor 1973; Wood 1973; Gross 1982; Nakagawara 1988):

(1) plant environment survey;

(2) vision screening;

(3) implementation of the programme;

(4) maintenance of the programme.

Plant environment survey

Initially, the potential hazards of the plant should be assessed. For example, there may be acids, flying particles from a lathe, or radiation from welding, against which the eyes need to be protected. The area of the plant and any particular dangerous task should be noted. Once the hazard has been identified, a method of eliminating or controlling it must be devised. Hazards may be eliminated at their source by modifying the design of the machinery or equipment, and the layout of the work place. In some circumstances non-hazardous materials may be used instead of the original hazardous ones. If the hazard cannot be eliminated then it must be controlled or contained. Screens or splash guards can be fitted around machines; exhaust systems installed to remove dust, gases or fumes from the atmosphere; and water sprays can be used to reduce the problems of dust in the atmosphere (Collins 1983). The wearing of eye protectors should be the last option. If eye protectors are required then the areas where they should be worn must be clearly marked.

There is little doubt that poor lighting can be a contributory factor in some accidents. Lighting conditions should be assessed for the various tasks to check that they are appropriate for the job to be performed efficiently. In the UK the CIBS code (1984) gives recommended lighting levels for various tasks and industries; this should be consulted.

Sites of emergency first aid equipment should be noted and the need for any additional equipment and their placement should also be assessed. For example, where chemicals are being used, a water fountain or shower unit should be installed to provide rapid dousing with water to dilute any chemicals accidentally splashed on an employee.

Accident records from the factory first aid centre can be analysed to determine where and how ocular injuries have occurred. A note should always be made of whether eye protectors were being worn at the time of injury and, if not, whether they should have been. This information can be very useful in determining areas where injuries are likely to occur and in investigating their causes to prevent any further injuries.

Vision screening

The visual efficiency of the employees is one aspect that is often neglected. Various studies have shown that about one-third of employees have vision below the standard required for their occupation and there has been a considerable amount of research supporting the relationship between accidents and defective vision. For example, one study cited by Grundy (1981), found that when vision screening was carried out in a large steel works, employees whose vision was below the standard required were found to have experienced on average 20 per cent more accidents than those who were visually efficient. Obviously, an employee whose vision is below standard is more likely to sustain self-injuries and to injure colleagues. Methods of assessing the visual efficiency of the employees may be carried out using a screening method, as described in Chapter 2 (see p. 24). Vision screening can be carried out to detect those employees whose vision is not up to the vision standard required. Employees found to have a visual defect can then be referred to a qualified person for further investigation. Fortunately, the majority of cases can be corrected, given appropriate professional advice and correct treatment.

Implementation

It is important that the eye protection programme is carried out correctly; incorrect administration could result in a work environment that is more hazardous than that found initially. Depending on the findings of the plant survey the following actions may be necessary:

1. Elimination or control of ocular hazards.

2. Provision of eye protectors. These must be personally issued to make sure that they fit correctly and they must be the correct type for the task involved.

3. Areas where ocular hazards exist, and where eye protection must be worn, should be marked clearly. They may be designated by lines painted on the floor or by warning signs placed in prominent positions. Since 1 January 1986 all new UK work place signs must comply with BS 5378 (1980) Part 1. This standard divides safety signs and notices into four categories, according to the type of message: (i) prohibition; (ii) mandatory;

(iii) warning; and (iv) safe condition. Each category has its own distinctive shape and colour (Fig. 3.3). Provisions must be made for eye protectors to be readily available for visitors to the hazardous areas.

4. First aid facilities. These should be set up so that immediate medical attention can be provided. All employees should be made aware of the first aid centres, and they should be clearly signposted. Other emergency equipment that is required in hazardous work areas should be easily accessible, for example water fountains in chemical factories.

5. Lens cleaning stations should be made available. These should contain cleaning solutions, anti-fog solutions, and clean cloths with which to wipe the eye protectors. Such stations are necessary to prevent cleaning with the first means available to the employee, often an oily rag. This will smear the lenses, making matters worse not better and the employee may then remove the eye protectors to see more clearly, leaving the eyes unprotected.

6. A safety committee be formed, which includes employee representatives.

7. Employees should be educated about the hazards involved in their jobs and the need for eye protection. Films, posters, and lectures, especially concerning the ocular consequences of failing to use eye protection, are very useful in impressing the importance of wearing eye protectors where necessary. There is a great need to motivate employees to wear their eye protection (Wigglesworth 1970), and employees should be made aware of their legal obligations concerning the wearing of eye protectors. In the UK the Royal Society for the Prevention of Accidents (RoSPA) provides safety films, posters, and lectures, all of which are extremely useful.

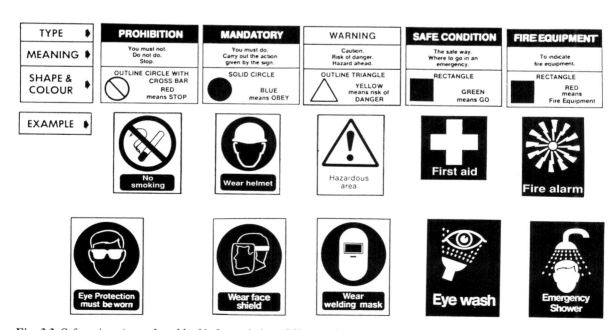

Fig. 3.3 Safety signs (reproduced by kind permission of Signs and Labels Ltd, Stockport, Cheshire).

Explanations of the initial symptoms that may be experienced when wearing eye protectors, especially by non-spectacle wearers should be given. Problems such as a restricted field of view, reflection and aberrations from the lenses, and magnification, should be discussed.

Accident record sheets should be kept at the first aid centre. Anyone requiring treatment should have the following details recorded (Rooke *et al.* 1980; Collins 1983):

(1) how the injury occurred;

(2) the cause of the accident;

(3) where the injury occurred;

(4) whether eye protection being worn and if it should have been, but was not, why not?

(5) the mechanical condition of the machine or tools used;

(6) apparent injury to eye;

(7) time and date of injury.

It is important to avoid suggesting blame in the questions. The above information is necessary for several reasons:

1. Insurance purposes and any claims for compensation by the employee.

2. Accident data collection and analysis.

3. A re-evaluation of the eye protection programme.

Maintenance of the programme

The maintenance of the programme is essential for continued safety and cost-effectiveness. It may involve:

1. Assessing new manufacturing processes and their potential hazards.

2. Continuing education and training for the employees.

3. Maintenance of lens cleaning and first aid facilities.

4. Vision screening, which should be carried out at regular intervals to maintain the necessary standard of vision.

5. Maintaining an active safety committee so that the employees can suggest methods of improving the safety of their environment.

6. Maintenance of stocks of replacement eye protectors. Employees should be informed as to the location of these supplies, which should be readily available. Any adjustments to the fitting of the eye protectors should be carried out by trained personnel to provide maximum comfort and protection. Frame heaters, screwdrivers, etc. should be available for the adjustment and maintenance of the eye protectors.

7. Recognition of employee achievements regarding their efforts to maintain and create a safer environment.

Summary

There are far too many eye injuries, which can have devastating results. Injuries occur at all ages, at home, at work or during leisure activities; unfortunately an alarmingly high number involve children. There is a need for people to be made aware of the potential ocular hazards and the necessity to wear eye protection. The optometrist can play an important educative and clinical role in the provision of eye protection. Advice can be given regarding the visual abilities and safety of the employees in relation to the particular job requirements. Assessing the working conditions and, where necessary, making recommendations for improvement are also part of the optometrist's role in preventive eye care.

References

BS 5378 Part 1 (1980). *Safety signs and colours — specification for colour and design.* British Standards Institution, London.

Canavan, Y.M., O'Flaherty, J., Archer, D.B., and Elwood, J.H. (1980). A 10 year survey of eye injuries in Northern Ireland 1967–76. *Br. J. Ophthalmol.*, **64**, 618–25.

Chiapella, A.P. and Rosenthal, A.R. (1985). One year in an eye casualty clinic. *Br. J. Ophthalmol.*, **69**, 865–70.

CIBS (1984). *Code for interior lighting.* The Chartered Institution of Building Services, London.

Cole, M.D., Clearkin, L., Dabbs, T., and Smerdon, D. (1987). The seat belt law and after. *Br. J. Ophthalmol.*, **71**, 436–40.

Collins, M. (1983). *Occupational public health optometry.* Queensland Institute of Technology, Queensland, Australia.

Easterbrook, M. (1981). Eye injuries in racket sports: a continuous problem. *Physician and Sportsman*, **9**(1), 91–9.

Easterbrook, M. (1988). Ocular injuries in racquet sports. *Int. Ophthal. Clinics*, **28**(3), 232–7.

Farmer, D. (1982). Eye protection bought into perspective. *Health and Safety at Work*, **April**, 20–4.

Freeman, H.M. (ed.) (1979). *Ocular trauma* p. 360. Prentice Hall International Inc, London.

Gervais, G. (1989). Patient resistance to the wearing of safety spectacles, B.Sc. Final year project, Department of Optometry, U.W.C.C., Cardiff.

Giovinazzo, V.J., Yannuzzi, L.A., Sorenson, J.A., Delrowe, D.J., and Cambell, E.A. (1987). The ocular complications of boxing. *Ophthalmol. (Rochester)*, **94**, 587–97.

Gregg, J.R. (1987). *Vision and sports — an introduction.* Butterworth–Heinemann, Stoneham, MA.

Gregory, P.T.S. (1986). Sussex Eye Hospital sports injuries. *Br. J. Ophthalmol.*, **70**, 748–50.

Gross, A. (1982). How the Norfolk and Western Railway drastically reduced the on the job injuries. *Sightsaving*, **51**, 14–17.

Grundy, J.W. (1981). Eyes geared for the job. *Optical World*, **Dec**, 10–11.

Hall, N.F., Denning, A.M., Elkington, A.R., and Cooper, P.J. (1985). The eye and seat belt wear in Wessex. *Br. J. Ophthalmol.*, **69**, 317–19.

Health and Safety Executive (1988). *Health and safety statistics 1985–1986.* HMSO, London.

John, G., Witherspoon, C.D., Feist, R.M., and Morris, R. (1988). Ocular lawn mower injuries. *Ophthalmology*, **95**, 1367–70.

Johnson, P.B. and Armstrong, M.F.J. (1986). Eye injuries in Northern Ireland two years after seat belt legislation. *Br. J. Ophthalmol.*, **70**, 460–2.

Jones, N.P. (1988). One year study of severe eye injuries in sport. *Eye*, **2**, 484–7.

Kelly, S.P. (1987) Serious eye injuries in badminton players. *Br. J. Ophthalmol.*, **71**, 746–7.

Lambah, P. (1968). Adult injuries at Wolverhampton. *Trans. Ophthal. Soc. (UK)*, **88**, 661.

La Roche, G.R., McIntyre, L. and Schertzer, R.M. (1988). Epidemiology of severe eye injuries in childhood. *Ophthalmology*, **95**, 1603–7.

Lathey, M. (1973). Introduction of an eye protection programme. *Aust. J. Optom.*, **56**, 321–6.

Leventhal, H., Safer, M., and Panagis, D. (1983). Impact of communications on the self regulation of health beliefs, decisions and behaviour. *Health Education Quarterly*, **10**, 3–29.

MacEwen, C.J. (1989). Eye injuries: a prospective survey of 5671 cases. *Br. J. Ophthalmol.* **73**, 888–94.

Mills, N. (1985). Sports eye injuries—dimming the stars. *Sightsaving*, **54**(1), 2–7.

Moore, M.C. and Worthly, D.A. (1977). Ocular injuries in squash players. *Aust. J. Ophthalmol.*, **5**, 46.

Moore, A.T., McCartney, A., and Cooling, R.J. (1987). Ocular injuries associated with the use of airguns. *Eye*, **1**, 422–9.

Nakagawara, Van B. (1988). Functional model of an eye protection program: guide for the clinical optometrist. *J. Am. Optom. Assoc.*, **59**, 925–8.

National Society for the Prevention of Blindness (1980). *Vision problems in the US*. NSPB, New York.

National Society for the Prevention of Blindness (1984). *21 questions on eye safety*. NSPB, New York.

Parver, L.M. (1988). The national eye trauma system. *Int. Ophthalmol.*, **28**, 203–5.

Powell, P., Hale, M., and Simon, M. (1971). *2,000 accidents: a shop floor study based on 42 months continuous observation*. National Institute of Industrial Psychology, London.

Randall, K.A. (1985). First aid for home eye injuries. *Sightsaving*, **54**(1), 10–14.

Rooke, F.C.E., Rothwell, P.J., and Woodhouse, D.F. (1980). *Ophthalmic nursing —its practice and management*, pp. 75–7. Churchill Livingstone, London.

Rosenstock, I., Derryberry, M., and Carriger, B.K. (1959). Why people fail to seek poliomyelitis vaccination. *Public Health Reports (UK)*, **74**, 98–103.

Taylor, H.A. (1973). Maintenance of an eye protection programme. *Aust. J. Optom.*, **56**, 86–90.

US CSPC (1983). *Estimated sports related eye injuries, selected sports*. Consumer Safety Product Commission. National Information Injury Clearing-house. Bethesda, Maryland.

Vinger, P.F. (1980). Sports-related eye injury. A preventable problem. *Surv. Ophthalmol.*, **25**(1), 47–51.

Vinger, P.F. (1985). Setting performance standards for sports eye guards. *Sightsaving*, **54**(1), 8–9.

Wigglesworth, E.C. (1970). Motivation in eye protection programs. *Am. J. Optom. A.A.A.O.*, **47**(2), 891–8.

Wood, K.H. (1973). Introduction of an eye protection programme. *Aust. J. Optom.*, **56**, 63–9.

Woods, T.A. (1988). The role of opticianry in preventing ocular injury. *Int Ophthal. Clinics*, **28**(3), 251–4.

Wykes, W.N. (1988). A 10-year survey of penetrating eye injuries in Gwent, 1976–85. *Br. J. Ophthalmol.*, **72**, 607–11.

Further reading

Gregg, J.R. (1987). *Vision and sports—an introduction*. Butterworth–Heinemann, Stoneham, MA.

Nylman, J.S. (ed.) (1989). *Problems in optometry. Ocular emergencies. Vol 1. No. 1.* J.B. Lippincott Company, Philadelphia.

Videos

Eyes in Industry. Health & Safety Executive. Available from C.F.L. Vision, Po Box 35, Wetherby, West Yorkshire.

Look out—Eye protection. RoSPA and The Two Rons.

IS 343, The RoSPA Film Library, Cannon House, The Priory Queensway, Birmingham.

4. Ocular injuries—mechanical*

Chapter 3 outlined the causes and frequency of eye injuries and this chapter will discuss the resultant effects upon the eye. Eye injuries, whatever their cause and however minor they appear to be, should always be treated seriously. All are potentially dangerous because of the possibility of infection or other secondary effects.

Ocular hazards can be divided into two main groups: mechanical and non-mechanical (Fig. 4.1).

The effects of these hazards upon the eye are numerous and have been described in depth by several books (see Further reading). Mechanical injuries may arise from a variety of causes. Their effects are generally divided into two main categories:

(1) contusion;
(2) perforation.

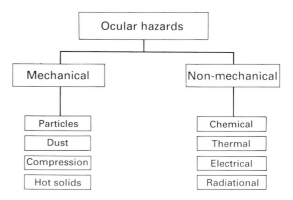

Fig. 4.1 Classification of ocular hazards.

* The main references used in compiling this chapter are Duke-Elder (1972) and Fox (1973).

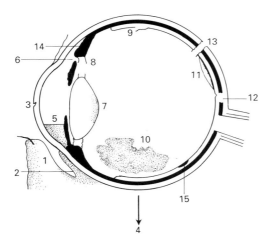

Fig. 4.2 Composite diagram of the possible ocular effects of a contusion injury (modified from Coakes and Holmes Sellors 1985 and courtesy of Butterworth–Heinemann (Oxford) Ltd). 1, black eye; 2, subconjunctival haemorrhage; 3, corneal abrasion; 4, blow-out fracture; 5, hyphaema; 6, iridodiaysis; 7, cataract; 8, lens subluxation due to torn zonule; 9, retinal tear/detachment; 10, vitreous haemorrhage; 11, commotio retinae; 12, choroidal rupture; 13, scleral rupture; 14, angle recession; 15, retinal haemorrhage.

Contusion injuries

Contusion injuries may result from a variety of causes, e.g. flying blunt objects (for example a squash ball), falling objects, the employee falling, explosions or compressed air accidents, fluid under pressure escaping from burst pipes, or water jets from fire hoses (Acheson *et al.* 1987; Noble and McFazdean 1987).

The resultant ocular damage is due to a wave of pressure traversing the fluid content of the eye. As the fluid is incompressible the blow will act as an explosive force in all directions from the centre outwards, resulting in the ocular contents being flung against their outer coat. The globe expands around the equator to take up a vertically oval shape. The effects of contusion on the various structures are numerous, and will now be discussed. Figure 4.2 shows some of the possible ocular injuries which may occur.

The eyelids and orbit

Eyelids—black eye

Fortunately, the eyes have their own natural defence: they are deeply set in bony orbits and have a fast blink reflex. Hence, the eye often escapes damage and the orbits and lids take the force of the blow. This frequently results in the appearance of a 'black eye'. Due to the vascularity and loose connective tissue structure of the lid, oedema and subcutaneous haemorrhages are common and usually occur rapidly after trauma. Haemorrhages may also spread under the conjunctiva, resulting in the lids being swollen and tightly shut. To examine the eye, the lids may need to be opened forcibly. A 'black eye' may spread to the other eye within 24 h as a result of subcutaneous blood infiltration (Fox 1973). The swelling and discoloration of the skin normally resolve within 2 weeks.

In more severe cases the haemorrhages may be due to intracranial damage. Such haemorrhages become apparent after 12–24 h, which is the time it takes for the blood to seep to the eyelids and forehead. This is a serious condition and X-rays must be taken to see whether there are fractures of the orbital bones.

Ptosis

Trauma to the upper lid may cause it to 'droop', which narrows the palpebral aperture. This is known as ptosis and may be caused by the lid being oedematous. In more severe cases there can be damage to the 3rd nerve, which supplies the levator muscle, or detachment of the muscle itself; the latter case will require surgery. Occasionally a 'partial protective' ptosis, or a tendency for the lid to close, will develop if there is an irritant causing discomfort and photophobia.

Ectropion

Damage to the lower lid may result in ectropion, a condition in which the lid margin turns away from the eye. This prevents the tears from draining properly through the puncta. Instead they flow down the cheek (epiphora) and can cause skin sores.

Fractures of the orbit

These can occur directly from a blow to the orbit or indirectly from radiating skull fractures. These injuries may also be associated with other facial fractures, head injuries, or severe lacerations.

Not surprisingly, the most common fracture affects the lateral wall of the orbit. The zygomatic bone and arch of the lateral wall may be fractured, resulting in depression of the lateral canthus and flattening of the cheek bone.

Fractures of the floor of the orbit may occur after a heavy blow and are known as blow-out fractures. The blow increases the intraorbital pressure, which causes the very thin bone of the maxilla to collapse into the maxillary sinus and the orbital contents then prolapse into the antrum. Elevation of the eye will be defective because the tissues surrounding the inferior rectus and inferior oblique muscle become trapped in the fracture (Fig. 4.3). Double vision will also be present in one or more directions of gaze. The herniation of the orbital contents results in a sinking or recession of the eye within the orbit (enophthalmos) with a narrowing of the palpebral fissure. There will also be loss of feeling on the same side of the face due to damage of the infraorbital nerve. Surgery, if required, should be carried out fairly promptly (within a week or two), before fibrous tissue has a chance to form. It will involve the insertion of a plate over the damaged orbital floor.

Damage to the nasal bone, ethmoidal sinuses and the medial wall is often apparent by the presence of air creptitus. Blowing the nose should be avoided, as air is forced under pressure into the soft tissue of the eyelids and surrounding skin, which results in swelling. As this can provide a

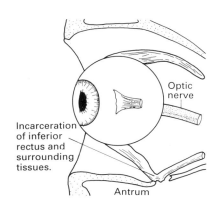

Fig. 4.3 Orbital floor fracture (after Elkington 1973*a*).

route for the spread of infection, a course of systemic antibiotics is usually given (Sachsenweger 1980).

Fractures of the superior orbital rim generally result in diplopia due to damage of the trochlear of the superior oblique muscle. This damage will be permanent unless there is early repair.

Inferior orbital rim damage is shown by ptosis or ectropion of the lower lid and by anaesthesia of infra-orbital nerve distribution. It is often associated with diplopia and hypotropia (Fox 1973).

Whenever a fracture is suspected, X-rays should be taken.

Anterior segment damage

Damage to the anterior segment may result in corneal abrasions, hyphaema and associated damage to the ciliary body, iris, or lens. Secondary complications, such as recurrent bleeding, uveitis, and abnormal intra-ocular pressure may also occur.

Subconjunctival haemorrhages

The conjunctiva, being the most superficial layer, often displays subconjunctival haemorrhages, but these reabsorb within several weeks and do not need treatment. However, subconjunctival haemorrhages caused by orbital bleeding can be so severe that the conjunctiva projects between the lids, and as mentioned above, requires prompt attention.

Hyphaema

The anterior chamber may appear red as the result of the presence of blood. This is known as hyphaema and is due to the rupture of a vessel in the iris or ciliary body. The chamber is generally only partially filled and the blood settles inferiorly. It will usually be reabsorbed without any serious consequences. However, in some cases, the anterior chamber may completely fill with blood (total hyphaema). If the blood is not reabsorbed after a few days, its colour changes from red to purple to black. This occurs due to a lack of oxygen from the aqueous and is sometimes referred to as an 'eight ball' hyphaema. This is a serious condition, as the intra-ocular pressure is generally elevated, resulting in secondary glaucoma and possible blood staining of the cornea.

Re-bleeding may occur, resulting in secondary glaucoma, blood-staining of the cornea, and permanent loss of vision. The source is uncertain, but it may arise from newly formed capillaries in the area of damage, or from the original leaking blood vessel. It usually occurs in the first five days after injury (Read and Goldberg 1974). Surgery is frequently required in cases of re-bleeding, and it should therefore be prevented if at all possible (Thomas et al. 1986). Given the possible complications, hyphaemas must always be referred, however small the amount of blood visible in the anterior chamber. The individual may be admitted to hospital and bed rest given for a couple of days. Hyphaemas may also indicate the presence of scleral ruptures. The most common sites are in a circumferential arc parallel to the corneal limbus, opposite to the impact site at either the insertion of rectus muscles on the globe or at the equator of the globe. This type of injury commonly occurs after a squash ball has hit the eye.

Iris

Damage to the iris may result in dilation or constriction of the pupil, this is known as traumatic mydriasis or traumatic miosis, respectively. Depending on the severity of the blow, the paralysis may be temporary, last only a few days, or permanent (Fox 1973).

Ruptures may occur to the sphincter pupillae, leaving a permanently irregular, semi-dilated pupil, which will not react to light or accommodation. The iris can be torn from its insertion to the ciliary body; this is known as iridodialysis. It is a permanent condition, usually accompanied by hyphaema, and results in a distortion of the pupil. Both conditions will cause symptoms of glare, especially in the case of iridodialysis where a second pupil has formed.

Angle recession

Traumatic angle recession of the anterior chamber can lead to the development of unilateral glaucoma months or years later. It is caused when the ciliary body has been torn from the sclera. Extensive angles of recession have been found in subjects with prolonged primary hyphaemas. The site of the recession can be predicted from the presence of traumatic mydriasis. The affected area of the pupil is atonic, neither fully dilates nor constricts, and corresponds to the position of the angle recession (Eagling 1974).

Lens

The zonular fibres that attach the lens to the ciliary body can be torn in a contusion injury. As a result, the lens may have become totally dislocated from its attachment, or partially dislocated (subluxated). The dislocated lens may fall either posteriorly into the vitreous, where low-grade ophthalmitis may occur, or enter the anterior chamber, causing corneal endothelial damage. There will be a marked hyperopic shift in the refraction and a tremulous iris (iridodonesis) may be seen due to the loss of support by the lens.

A subluxated lens produces a prismatic effect upon vision, with the upward displacement of objects. This may cause symptoms such as diplopia, nausea, and vomiting.

The sudden compression and expansion of the lens, with or without rupture of the capsule, can produce a cataract. In fact trauma is the most common cause of unilateral cataract in the young (Kanski 1984). Various types of lens changes which can occur, have been listed by Duke-Elder (1972) as:

(1) vossius ring opacity;

(2) sub-epithelial disseminated opacities;

(3) traumatic rosette-shaped cataract;

(4) diffuse cataract;

(5) zonular cataract.

VOSSIUS RING OPACITY

A circle of iris pigment known as the vossius ring may be seen on the lens after impaction of the iris. This usually occurs only in the young, as older, more sclerosed lenses will not accept such an imprint. The pigment is usually absorbed and may be replaced by fine capsular dots, which gradually clear later in life.

SUB-EPITHELIAL DISSEMINATED OPACITIES
The lens may appear to have small, discrete punctate or flake-like opacities, which lie beneath the anterior epithelium. These opacities may be transient, disappearing within a few days or weeks, or permanent. Occasionally, the development of these opacities is delayed, and they may not become apparent until several years after injury.

TRAUMATIC ROSETTE-SHAPED CATARACT
The rosette-shaped opacity may occur anteriorly or posteriorly and the onset may be delayed, in which case the opacities are usually found in the deeper cortical layers or the nucleus. This type of cataract may occur after perforating, as well as contusion types of injury.

DIFFUSE CATARACT
A diffuse concussion cataract is rare and is usually associated with a tear of the lens capsule. If the tear is large the lens fibres may spill into the anterior or posterior chamber. This will result in secondary glaucoma or an inflammation of the iris and ciliary body (anterior uveitis).

ZONULAR CATARACT
Zonular (lamellar) cataracts are rare and consist of a series of concentric, thin sheets of opacities surrounded by clear lens. They usually occur after extensive disseminated opacities or after rosette-shaped opacities.

Posterior segment damage
Damage to the posterior segment may initially be obscured from direct view by a hyphaema. The damage that may occur to the retina after contusion has been listed by Duke-Elder (1972) as:

(1) oedema, macula cysts and holes, necrosis, atrophic retinal changes;
(2) vascular changes—haemorrhages (embolism, thrombosis, aneurysm);
(3) tears of the choroid and retina;
(4) retinal detachment.

OEDEMA, CYSTS, HOLES, AND NECROSIS
The retina may appear milky-white within a few hours of the trauma and vision will be reduced. *Commotio retinae* is the term used to describe oedema of the retina; it is transient and reversible. The oedema usually subsides within 4 days and vision returns to normal. (Some authorities believe that the white retinal appearance is not due to oedema but to the derangement of the photoreceptors, whilst others believe it may be due to choroidal ischaemia; Deutsch and Feller 1985.) In some cases vision may be permanently impaired due to the development of pigmentary changes at the macula or to the formation of a macula cyst or hole. In severe injuries intraretinal haemorrhages or haemorrhages into the anterior vitreous from the pars plana region may occur.

VASCULAR CHANGES

Eyes with pathologically altered blood vessels, e.g. with hypertension, arteriosclerosis, or diabetes, are particularly vulnerable to haemorrhages. These haemorrhages may be retinal, subretinal, preretinal, or into the vitreous. They may cause a sudden and profound loss of vision and leave the site of retinal pathology obscured from view.

TEARS

Although the choroid is firmly attached to the sclera, choroidal tears are common and generally occur between the disc and macula, or temporal to the macula. They are cresentic, vertical, and of variable length; they may be single or multiple. Haemorrhages into the choroid, subretinal space, or the retina itself may occur after such tears. These haemorrhages are usually absorbed, leaving yellowish grey lesions in the choroid. The tears affect vision only if they are between the disc and macula. In one report only 39 per cent of patients with choroidal and retinal lesions from contusion injuries regained a visual acuity of 6/12 or better (Archer and Canavan 1983). A recent study by De Laey (1987) has noted that a late complication of choroidal ruptures may be choroidal neovascularization. This can usually be treated successfully by photocoagulation.

Choroidal detachment does not occur unless trauma is combined with decreased intra-ocular pressure. This allows fluid to pass into the suprachoroidal space, facilitating the detachment.

RETINAL DETACHMENT

This is the separation of the retina from the pigment epithelium, which may occur gradually or suddenly. In cases of a gradual detachment, the individual may be unaware of the condition, but such symptoms as floaters and photopsia (light flashes) due to vitreous traction on the retina may be experienced. Typically, if the retinal detachment occurs shortly after trauma, a peripheral retinal tear is found, frequently in the upper temporal region (Perkins and Hansell 1971). People with predisposing factors, such as myopia, peripheral retinal degeneration, and aphakia, where there are areas of retinal weakness, are more prone to retinal tears and hence detachments.

Scleral ruptures have been noted to occur after a severe blunt trauma and are commonly seen in the superior and anterior portions of the globe (Russel et al. 1988).

Nervous supply

The innervation to the eye may be affected after a contusion injury. Contusion of the infra-orbital nerve will lead to decreased sensitivity or anaesthesia of the skin in the area of distribution of the nerve. The infra-orbital nerve is damaged most frequently after blunt trauma, whereas the supra-orbital nerve is usually only affected after a sharp blow (Fox 1973).

The innervation to the extra-ocular muscles, which are responsible for eye movements, may also be affected. Horizontal double vision may occur due to 6th cranial nerve damage, but fortunately recovery is complete in most cases. If the 4th trochlear nerve is involved it gives rise to vertical double vision. Trauma to the 3rd nerve may result in mydriasis, ptosis, double vision, lack of adduction, and loss of accommodation. Traumatic hyperopia, due to the loss of accommodation, may be temporary or permanent. Myopic changes, which occur more commonly, are generally due to ciliary muscle spasm caused by irritation to the nerve or the muscle fibres. Myopic shifts in the order of 1–6 D may occur but in most cases they are transient and the refraction returns to normal within about a month (Duke-Elder 1972).

The optic nerve may be partially or completely ruptured, with partial or complete evulsion after blunt trauma (Noble and McFazdean 1987; Williams *et al.* 1987). Visual field defects will be found corresponding to the position of the damaged nerve fibres, so that there will be either partial or total loss of vision, depending on the severity of the injury; this loss of vision will be permanent. Papillitis, swelling of the optic disc, and optic atrophy following widespread retinal or choroidal damage, may also occur (Duke-Elder 1972).

Perforating injuries

Foreign bodies

This is the most common type of ocular trauma, accounting for about half of all types of injuries. It generally results from a person not realizing the hazard of the task, for instance when using a hammer and chisel, cutting wire, or grinding wheel. The eye's natural defence mechanisms may be penetrated and foreign bodies (FBs) may become embedded in the globe, or they may pass through the cornea or sclera to become lodged within the globe. The symptoms can vary from little or no discomfort to severe pain. Figure 4.4 shows the common sites of foreign bodies.

Subtarsal foreign bodies

Many small FBs will be washed out of the eye by the tears. Sometimes, however, the FB will become embedded in the subtarsal conjunctiva of the upper lid, which will cause pain on blinking and a vertical corneal

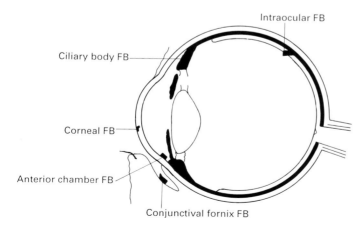

Fig. 4.4 Sites of ocular foreign bodies.

abrasion. The area of abraded cornea, where the epithelium has been removed, will be seen as a disturbance of the corneal reflection. This can be viewed by instilling fluorescein and viewing the eye under ultraviolet light. The upper lid must be everted if these FBs are to be located and removed. The healing of the epithelium may sometimes be incomplete, resulting in recurrent corneal erosions.

Superficial foreign bodies

An eye with a corneal FB usually shows marked vascular injection closest to its position (Novak 1970). Ocular pain will be experienced but it will be difficult to localize. If the corneal FB has been present for a couple of days a grey ring of infiltration may occur around it and, on removal, a small, pitted ulcer will remain. It may leave a permanent scar, although this will generally only affect vision if it is over the centre of the cornea. An FB embedded in the conjunctiva or sclera is often surrounded by haemorrhages.

According to Fox (1973) many FBs are metallic, iron particles being the most common, followed by copper and aluminium. The softer metals (e.g. magnesium) are a less frequent cause of FBs, as they tend to fragment less during drilling, sawing, grinding, or cutting. Metallic FBs left embedded in the eye will rapidly oxidize under the influence of the enzymes of the cornea and tears. This may set up a severe inflammation of the cornea or iris. The oxidation of steel is much faster than that of aluminium or magnesium, and a rust ring may be apparent within a couple of hours. A rust deposit left in the cornea will partially dissolve and an iron stain will diffuse into stromal or subepithelial layers.

Intra–ocular foreign bodies

The possible presence of an intra–ocular foreign body (IOFB) should always be investigated, especially when the symptoms are a gush of fluid from the eye with blurring of vision. Small, hot FBs hitting the eye at great speed may penetrate the globe and actually seal their route of entry. As only a slight pain is experienced, it is essential not to miss an IOFB, as it may lead to loss of vision. Whenever the eye is perforated an X-ray should be taken to exclude the presence of a metallic IOFB. The classic signs of a perforating injury are a shallow anterior chamber, eccentricity of the pupil, and prolapse of the iris. However, care must be taken in the following two cases (Elkington 1973a):

1. A small conjunctival haemorrhage, while being the only clue, may obscure deeper scleral laceration.
2. The eye appears normal but there is a history suggestive of an IOFB.

The IOFB may have been stopped by the iris and then fallen down into the anterior chamber angle to be hidden from view. If an IOFB has penetrated through the vitreous, fibrous tissue will form along its path. The fibrous tissue may impair vision if it crosses over the visual axis and a vitrectomy may then be required to restore vision and/or to prevent tractional retinal detachment.

There are various methods of localizing IOFBs: X-ray techniques, ultrasonography, binocular indirect ophthalmoscopy, and the use of a Berman and Roper Hall localizer, which employs electric induction currents (Deutsch and Feller 1985). Ultrasonography can locate the position of non-metallic fragments, whereas X-ray show metallic FB positions. Ultrasonography traces the rebound of high frequency pulsations and, by studying the resulting patterns, the inside of the eye can be explored. Once the IOFB has been located it can be removed.

Retained intra-ocular foreign bodies

Vegetable FBs may cause infections so severe that a purulent panophthalmitis may occur in only a few hours. According to Fox (1973), other FBs may be retained without noticeable reaction, e.g. gold, silver, platinium, glass, and many plastics. Less well tolerated by the eye are lead, zinc, nickel, and aluminium particles. These are often coated in an inert salt and later encapsulated by a fibrous tissue coating, rendering them less toxic. The most dangerous IOFBs are iron and copper, which cause siderosis and chalcosis, respectively. In siderosis the iron oxidizes and causes a slow, insidious intra-ocular reaction as it permeates most of the ocular tissues (Elkington 1973a); this can lead to complete blindness. It is a late-occuring syndrome and the ferrous pigmentation causes a rusty coloration of the cornea, iris, or lens. In addition, a series of chronic degenerative changes occur, which lead to pupil dilation because of atrophy of the sphincter pupillae, cataract, and then retinal detachment and open angle glaucoma. These complications usually occur between 2 months and 2 years after injury, and surgery is needed immediately after injury to remove the foreign body (Deutsch and Feller 1985).

Pure copper will cause a rapid inflammation of the eye (chalcosis) and the eye may be lost if endophthalmitis occurs. Copper alloys (bronze and brass) may induce chronic degenerative processes by slow diffusion of the copper, which tends to be taken up by the limiting membranes of the eye (Elkington 1973a). A green ring may develop in the peripheral cornea in Descemet's membrane (Kayser–Fleisher ring) and a sunflower cataract in the anterior capsule of the lens is formed. It is not usually as essential to remove copper as iron IOFBs, as retained particles may not cause a significant loss of vision for many years.

Another complication after IOFB trauma has been noted by Trimble and Schatz (1986), who reported cases where subretinal neovascularization occurred 6–8 months after a metallic IOFB. This was successfully treated by photocoagulation.

Lacerations

In cases where lacerations involve the cornea and sclera, there may be a prolapse of the iris, ciliary body, lens, and vitreous, resulting in complete disorganization of the globe. Posterior rupture of the globe is rare and should be suspected when extreme conjunctival oedema and haemorrhage with marked hypotony occur. Unfortunately, useful vision is not often restored, even after prompt surgery. Lacerations may also occur after blunt trauma; for example, two cases of lacerations caused by jets of water from an agricultural sprinkler have been reported (Salminen and Ranta 1983).

Infections of the eye

The danger of IOFBs is that they may carry infections into the eye, resulting in uveitus—inflammation of the entire uveal tract. Infections may be caused by brucellosis or toxoplasmosis (McWilliam 1973). This is not as serious as a purulent infection, which usually results in the loss of the eye due to panophthalmitis or endophthalmitis.

A very rare and serious complication of perforating lacerations from an IOFB is sympathetic ophthalmitis, a type of uveitis affecting the non-injured eye, and which can lead to blindness. The second eye usually becomes involved 2 weeks to 2 months after injury (Elkington 1973b). According to a recent review the only effective therapy is preventive enucleation of the injured eye despite the use of immunosuppressive agents (Albert and Diaz-Rohena 1989).

An individual who has received a perforating injury should be sent for immediate medical attention. The eye should never be padded, as this may cause the ocular contents to prolapse. A cardboard cone can be placed over the eye to protect it from dust, dirt, etc. X-rays should be taken if the presence of an IOFB is suspected, to determine if it is metallic.

To summarize, contusion and perforating injuries are the most common causes of ocular trauma. The extent of the injuries can be minor or very severe and a person with an eye injury requires medical attention to assess the situation and the treatment needed.

References

Acheson, J.F., Wong, D., and Chignell, A.H. (1987). Eye injuries caused by direct jets of water from a fire hose. *Br. Med. J.*, **292**, 481–2.

Albert, D.M. and Diaz-Rohena, R. (1989). A historical review of sympathetic ophthalmia and its epidemiology. *Surv. Ophthal.*, **34**, 1–14.

Archer, D.B. and Canavan, Y.M. (1983). Contusional eye injuries: retinal and choroidal lesions. *Aust. J. Ophthalmol.*, **11**, 251–64.

Coakes, R.L. and Holmes Sellors, P.J. (1985). *An outline of ophthalmology*. Wright and Sons Ltd., Bristol.

De Laey, J.J. (1987). Choroidal neovascularisation after traumatic choroidal rupture. *Bull. Soc. Belge. Ophthalmol.*, **220**, 53–9.

Deutsch, T.A. and Feller, D.B. (1985). *Paton and Goldberg's management of ocular injuries*, (2nd edn). W.B. Saunders & Co., Philadelphia, PA.

Duke-Elder, S. (ed.) (1972). *System of ophthalmology—injuries*, Vol. XIV, Parts 1 & 2. S. Duke-Elder and P.A. MacFaul. Henry Kimpton, London.

Eagling, E.M. (1974). Ocular damage after blunt trauma to the eye—its relationship to the nature and extent of the injury. *Br. J. Ophthalmol.*, **58**, 126–39.

Elkington, A.R. (1973a). Intraocular foreign bodies. *Nursing Times*, **Dec**, 1638–9.

Elkington, A.R. (1973b). Perforating wounds. *Nursing Times*, **Nov**, 1597–8.

Fox, S.L. (1973). *Industrial and occupational ophthalmology*. C.C. Thomas, IL.

Kanski, J.J. (1984). *Clinical ophthalmology*. Butterworths, London.

McWilliams, R.J. (1973). Infection of the eye. *Nursing Times*, **Feb**, 145–6.

Noble, M.J. and McFazdean, R. (1987). Indirect injury to the optic nerve and optic chiasm. *Neuro. Ophthalmol.*, **7**, 341–8.

Novak, J.F. (1970). Ocular trauma in industry. *J. Occup. Med.*, **12**, 287–90.

Perkins, E.S. and Hansell, P. (1971). *An atlas of diseases of the eye*, (2nd. edn.) Churchill Livingston, London.

Read, J. and Goldberg, M.F. (1974). Blunt ocular trauma and hyphema. *Int. Ophthal. Clin.*, **14**, 57–9.

Russel, S.R., Olsen, K.R., and Folk, J.C. (1988). Predictors of scleral rupture and the role of vitrectomy in severe blunt ocular trauma. *Am. J. Ophthalmol.*, **105**, 253–7.

Sachsenweger, R. (1980). *Illustrated handbook of ophthalmology*. Wright and Son Ltd, Bristol.

Salminen, L. and Ranta, A. (1983). Orbital laceration caused by a blast of water: report of two cases. *Br. J. Ophthalmol.*, **67**, 840–1.

Thomas, M.A., Parrish, R.K. II, and Feuer, W.J. (1986). Rebleeding after traumatic hyphema. *Arch. Ophthalmol.*, **104**, 206–10.

Trimble, S.N. and Schatz, H. (1986). Subretinal neovascularisation following metallic intraocular foreign body trauma. *Arch. Ophthalmol.*, **104**, 515–19.

Williams, D.F., Williams, G.A., Abrams, G.W., Jesmanowicz, A., and Hyde, J.S. (1987). Evulsion of the retina associated with optic nerve evulsion. *Am. J. Ophthalmol.*, **104**, 5–9.

Further reading

Deutsch, T.A. and Feller, B. (Eds) (1985). *Paton and Goldberg's Management of ocular injuries*. W.B. Saunders, Philadephia.

Duke-Elder, S. (ed.) (1972). *System of ophthalmology—injuries*, Vol. XIV, Part 1 & 2. S. Duke-Elder and P.A. McFaul. Henry Kimpton, London.

Fox, S.L. (1973). *Industrial and occupational ophthalmology*. C.C. Thomas, Illinois.

Nyman, J.S. (ed.) (1989). *Problems in optometry. Ocular emergencies*, Vol. 1, No. 1. J.B. Lippincott, Philadelphia.

Roper-Hall, M.J. (1987). *Eye emergencies*. Churchill Livingstone, Edinburgh.

Shingleton, B.J., Hersh, P.S., and Kenyon, K.R. (1991). *Eye trauma*. Mosby-Year Book, St Louis.

5. Ocular injuries— non-mechanical[*]

The non-mechanical injuries fall into four main categories:

(1) chemical;
(2) thermal;
(3) electrical;
(4) radiational.

Chemical injuries

Most chemicals harm the eyes by direct contact with the external ocular tissues; these are amongst the most urgent ocular emergencies. Concentrated sulphuric acid from exploding car batteries, household bleaches, detergents, disinfectants, and lime are examples of chemicals that can cause burns to the eyes. However, it should not be forgotten that chemicals can also cause damage to the internal ocular structures, e.g. retina and optic nerve, through systemic absorption.

Direct effect of chemicals

The main groups of chemicals that produce damage, and that may be in the form of gas, vapour, liquid, or solid, are:

(1) acids;
(2) alkalis;
(3) organic solvents;
(4) surfactants;
(5) irritants and allergens;
(6) aerosols.

Acids

The severity of the burn depends on the concentration of the chemical, the duration of the exposure, and the pH of the solution. Inorganic acids

[*] Most of this section has been summarized from Duke-Elder (1972) and Fox (1973).

include sulphuric acid, nitric acid, and hydrochloric acid. When splashed, these acids may burn the eyelids and face, but fortunately the lid closure reflex is so fast that the eyeball is not generally affected. It may, however, suffer subsequently from exposure as a result of scar tissue formation and contraction of the lids. All solutions are irritating to the eye but rarely serious if their pH is 2.5 or above (Fox 1973). Diluted acids produce redness, oedema, and small conjunctival haemorrhages. Prolonged exposure causes ulceration and opaqueness of the cornea and conjunctival epithelium. The epithelium normally regenerates to leave a clear cornea. However, if the acid is strong, then stromal opacification and corneal vascularization will occur. The tissues may even be charred by concentrated nitric or sulphuric acids and, in the severest cases, complete destruction of the cornea and anterior structures will result.

The damage caused by acids depends upon the protein affinity of the acid anion and the concentration of the acid (Novak 1970). The acids act by combining chemically with the protein of the more superficial tissues to form an insoluble acid proteinate. This acts as a buffer, which limits the penetration of the acid through the tissues, cornea, etc.

Acid burns are generally less severe than alkali burns and they tend to improve with treatment and time. They are common in artificial silk manufacturing, as the viscous process exposes the workers to a fine spray of sulphuric acid. Acid burns are also frequently associated with glass injuries resulting from flasks and bottles breaking and there have been reports of exploding car batteries causing sulphuric acid burns to the eyes (Minatoya 1978).

In general, organic acids penetrate the cornea, only slightly and rarely cause dense corneal opacification. This group of acids includes formic, acetic, and citric acids (Duke-Elder 1972).

Alkalis

Alkalis penetrate tissues rapidly. They act by combining with the lipoid cells of the membranes and produce total disruption of cells with softening of the tissues (Deutsch and Feller 1985). Once the alkali has gained entry to the corneal stroma, it progresses to Descemet's membrane by the cations combining temporarily with the mucoproteins and collagen. The mucoproteins are then denatured rapidly and the released cations attach themselves to even deeper stromal proteins (Fox 1973). The initial appearance of the eye after trauma may be deceiving, showing little apparent damage, but it may become worse with time, leaving a totally opaque cornea.

Salts of weak acids and strong bases, such as sodium carbonate, and organic amines have strong alkaline reactions; phenols also act similarly to alkalis.

The ocular effects of alkalis have been studied and noted to progress through three stages (Hughes 1946; Brown *et al.* 1972):

1. Acute stage. Ischaemic necrosis of the conjunctiva; sloughing of the corneal epithelium; oedema; and opacification of the subconjunctival tissue, the substantia propria, and acute iritis.

2. Reparation stage. Epithelium regenerates, vascularization appears, and the iritis subsides.

3. Late complications. Symblepharon; an opaque, vascularized cornea with recurrent ulcerations; uveitis; secondary glaucoma; and cataract.

There is a rapid increase in the intra-ocular pressure after severe chemical burns, especially with alkalis. The mechanisms responsible for the increase in intra-ocular pressure are a temporary shrinkage of the corneal collagen (Paterson and Pfister 1974) and a breakdown of the blood aqueous barrier due to the lysis of the cells lining, and adjacent to, the anterior chamber. This causes intense exudation of cells, etc. into the anterior chamber, which may lead to a severe fibrinous inflammatory reaction in the conjunctiva as well as in the anterior chamber of the eye. This leads to the later complication of symblepharon, an adhesion between the bulbar and palpebral conjunctiva, and a dry eye.

As the hydroxyl ion concentration increases, the severity of the effects increases; a pH above 11 is exceedingly dangerous. However, as alkalis have different fat solubilities, the penetration ability of the cornea varies. Ammonium hydroxide has the greatest ability to dissolve fats and it penetrates the cornea rapidly, to produce deep injury. Other chemicals frequently involved in burns are the sodium, potassium, ammonium, and calcium hydroxides (Fox 1973). Lime burns are very serious and commonly occur in the building trades (Moon and Robertson 1983). Calcium oxide is a major ingredient of substances such as cement, lime, mortar, white-washes, and numerous other compounds used in this industry. When water or tears are added to calcium oxide heat is created, causing a thermal burn. In addition, calcium hydroxide is produced, which increases the damage to the eye. Lime in particular, tends to adhere to the cornea and conjunctiva and causes excessive lacrimation.

Experiments on rabbits by Brown *et al.* (1969) have shown that the corneal ulceration after an alkali burn is due to the collagenolytic enzyme produced by the cornea. This had led to the use of collagenase inhibitors, such as L-cysteine, in the treatment of alkali burns to reduce the corneal ulceration. Other types of treatment include the use of EDTA, ascorbic acid, and citric acid (Pfister 1983).

Organic solvents

Numerous substances of this type are used in various industries, but they rarely cause permanent damage. Exposure to their vapour causes irritation and a more intense reaction occurs if they are splashed into the eye as a liquid. They cause superficial punctate keratitis of the cornea and conjunctiva. Some of the compounds are caustic and may enter the stroma, denature the protein, and produce scarring. The subjective symptoms are pain, photophobia, lacrimation, and stinging. Such complaints are reported by those working with lacquers when solvents such as alcohol, acetone, camphor, ether, toluene, benzol, and acetates are used.

Table 5.1 lists the organic solvents, along with their uses in industry, as classified by Duke-Elder (1972).

It is also important to note that, when absorbed, these solvents have toxic effects that suppress the central nervous system.

Table 5.1 Classification of organic solvents and their uses (from Duke-Elder 1972)

Type of Organic solvent	Example	Industrial use
Hydrocarbons— aliphatic and aromatic	Benzene	In dyeing, leather, rubber, linoleum, paints, varnish and lacquer industries; motor fuels
Halogenated hydrocarbons	Trichloroethylene	Solvents for fats, waxes, gums, resins, oils. Used in rubber and cellulose industries and in manufacture of paints, lacquers and varnishes; insecticides; antiseptics
Alcohols	Ethanol	Solvents and used in lacquers and polishes
Ketones	Acetone	Solvent in plastics, rubber, dyes and paint industries
Aldehydes	Methyl aldehyde	Solvent for oils, resins, cellulose. Used in plastics and rubber industries
Ether	Ethylether	Solvent in plastics manufacture
Ester	Methyl formate	Solvent in many industries; it is the least toxic organic solvent

Surfactants

These compounds have a fat-soluble group at one end of the molecule and a water-soluble group at the other end. This structure allows the compound to lower the surface tension of water and to make fat-soluble materials miscible. They are used as industrial detergents and as emulsifying agents and cause contact dermatitis and mucosal irritation. Surfactants are divided into three main groups: (i) cationic; (ii) anionic; and (iii) non-ionic (Duke-Elder 1972; Fox 1973; Grant 1974). The cationic group of surfactants cause damage to the cornea and conjunctiva by precipitating the protein and, if severe enough, will lead to opacification of the corneal stroma, with subsequent vascularization; quaternary ammonium compounds, such as benzylkonium chloride, belong to this group. Anionic surfactants, such as soap, cause slow saponification of intracellular lipoid substances and lysis of the cells. Healing occurs quite quickly, leaving no permanent damage (Fox 1973). The non-ionic surfactants are usually esters of fatty acids with polyoxyethylene or sorbitol. These do not cause any permanent damage as any corneal erosions produced heal with no scarring.

Irritants and allergens

Numerous substances may irritate the eyes without causing permanent damage. A true allergy requires sensitization of cells by prior exposure to an allergen. Subsequent exposure to the allergen will then result in a typical allergic reaction. Common allergens are organic substances of animal or vegetable origin, e.g. wool, pollen, and dairy products. They produce the characteristic redness and swelling of tissues of the lids and conjunctiva.

As new processes are introduced into industry, the number of substances causing dermatitis and conjunctivitis increase, and many have not yet been isolated. Unfortunately the appearance of the skin and conjunctiva often give no clue to the actual agent involved.

It is possible to desensitize people who are liable to attacks. In certain industries, allergic skin reactions are well known and are recognized as industrial diseases. Special trades may have easily identifiable irritants but there is no explanation as yet for the fact that large numbers of people work for years with common irritants, such as soap, without any ill effects.

Industries with a high percentage of workers reporting dermatitis include baking, chemical manufacturing, engineering, metal working, painting, preserving, and textile manufacturing. Adequate ventilation and protective goggles should be provided where necessary to prevent dust and fumes contacting the eyes, as these may cause serious secondary effects, such as purulent conjunctivitis and corneal erosions.

Aerosols

Aerosols are commonly used in households as well as industry. Their fine spray can cause a superficial corneal inflammation, known as superficial punctate keratitis. After staining with fluorescein these show up quite clearly as small punctate dots when seen under ultraviolet (UV) light; these are temporary.

Indirect effects of chemicals

Chemicals come in various forms (solid, liquid, powder, dust, mist or vapour) and some can be toxic to the eye if they are accidentally ingested, absorbed, or inhaled. Neurotoxic agents, such as organic solvents and heavy metals and their salts and alcohols, can cause optic neuritis or other ocular toxicities. Many industrial poisons affect the eyes, and Table 5.2 shows the effects of some commonly used chemicals upon the ocular tissues (for further details see Grant 1974; Hunter 1975).

Treatment of chemical trauma

The ideal method of treatment is to neutralize the chemical. As this is often not possible, and as time may be lost looking for the appropriate solution, immediate and prolonged irrigation of the eye with water or

Table 5.2 Indirect effects of some commonly used chemicals

Structure	Effect	Chemical	Uses
Cornea and conjunctiva	Discoloration	Iron minerals, dinitrobenzene	Organic solvent
Cornea	Scarring	Hydroquinine	
	Deposits and opacities	Beryllium gold, silver, mercury	
	Anaesthesia	Carbon disulphide	Rayon/viscose
	Inflammation	Ethylbenzene	industry
Lens	Opacities	Dinitrophenol, naphthalene	Dye industry, insecticides
	Deposits and discoloration	Copper, mercury	
Anterior uveal tract	Iris atrophy	Quinine	
	Dilated pupil	Carbon monoxide, nitrous fumes	
	Constricted pupil and cilary body spasms	Parathion and lindane	Insecticides
Retina	Oedema	Cyanide, methanol	Solvent for shellacs
	Haemorrhages	Benzene, methyl bromide	Cleaning fluid, refrigerants and fire extinguishers
Optic nerve	Neuritis and atrophy	Lead, methanol, dinitrobenzol, trichloroethylene, carbon tetrachloride, carbon disulphide, benzene, methylbromide, naphthaline	Heavy metals, organic solvents
	Papilloedema	Benzene, lead	
	Pigment degeneration	Copper, iron	
Visual pathways	Cortical blindness	Carbon monoxide	
	Homonymous hemianopia	Lead	

Compiled from Duke-Elder (1972), Grant (1974), Hunter (1975), and Tier (1983).

saline should be carried out. The faster the chemical is diluted, the better the prognosis. Water fountains, showers, etc. should be available in areas where chemicals are being used so that accidental spills or splashes of chemicals can be dowsed immediately with water. Irrigation should be continued for at least 20 min and the eye should not be padded, so that the tears continue to wash out any residual chemical. Any chemical particles that remain should also be removed. Various solutions are recommended for lime, mortar, and plaster, including 11 per cent disodium

Table 5.3 Prognosis for eyes subjected to chemical burns

Appearance on initial examination	Prognosis	
	Acid	Alkali
Red eye—with or without corneal staining	Reasonably good	Uncertain
Cornea has a dull appearance, conjunctiva oedematous and limbal vessels obliterated.	Uncertain	Poor
White eye with coagulated necro... of the conjunctiva and cornea	Poor	Poor

edetate, 10 per cent ammonium tartrate, 10 per cent glucose solution (Porter 1966). For other alkali injuries, 2 per cent boric acid or 2 per cent acetic acid solutions are advised (Porter 1961). For acid burns, 3.5 per cent sodium bicarbonate solution is advised (O'Connor Davies 1981).

The injured employee should be referred to the casualty department of the local hospital for further irrigation. Treatment then depends on the severity of the burn. In mild cases it may involve the instillation of topical antibiotics to prevent secondary infection and a mydriatic to dilate the pupil. The use of topical steroids is controversial. Whilst they have a beneficial effect in reducing the inflammatory reaction, they can retard the repair processes and hence lead to corneal melting and perforation (Pfister 1983). In cases of alkali burns, citric acid has been shown to reduce the incidence of corneal ulceration in experiments by inhibiting polymorphs (Pfister *et al*. 1982). Collagenase inhibiting, such as L–cysteine, have also been reported to have a beneficial effect in preventing ulcers in alkali burned corneas (Brown *et al*. 1969). The fitting of a scleral contact lens may help prevent adhesions of the bulbar and palpebral conjunctiva, i.e. symblepharon. A full thickness corneal graft may be necessary if the cornea is opaque, but the prognosis is poor, especially if the cornea is vascularized (Morgan 1987).

Table 5.3 (Sachsenweger 1980) gives a summary of the prognosis for eyes affected by chemical burns depending on the appearance of the eye at the initial examination.

Thermal injuries

Thermal burns

There are two types of thermal burns: (i) flame; and (ii) contact burns. These may be caused by hot bodies, fluids, or gases. Burns usually involve the eye lids and not the globe, which will probably have been protected by the blink reflex. The characteristic picture is of marked oedema and tissue necrosis. In some cases it may be necessary to open the lids forcibly to inspect the globe and then provide treatment, if required.

Flame burns

These occur frequently and may result where high temperatures and inflammable liquids are being used. Gases, ovens, furnaces, and petrol stores are liable to explode, and soaked overalls are also a potential fire hazard. The eye is rarely involved unless the heat is so intense and prolonged that the lids are destroyed. Generally the lashes and brow are scorched and the lids may be burnt with extensive damage to the face, but the globe is unaffected. The burnt lids may need plastic surgery and ectropion must be prevented. There may be continuous weeping due to damaged lacrimal puncta and canaliculi, which have become blocked by subsequent fibrosis.

Contact burns

These may be caused by molten substances, such as metal or glass striking the cornea and entering the conjunctival sac. The molten substance solidifies as soon as it cools on hitting the eye and may fall into the lower fornix, where it continues to burn the surrounding tissue due to its latent heat. Prompt removal and irrigation reduces damage. The velocity of the hot particle may be such to perforate the eye, causing intra-ocular damage.

According to Duke Elder (1972), two different reactions may occur, depending on the temperature of the particle, its capacity to retain heat, and whether it is in solid or molten state. Glowing solid bodies that retain heat, i.e. slag, molten metal, or glass at temperatures of, say, 1000 °C cause severe burns, scarring of the cornea, and destruction of the conjunctiva, and this often leads to the loss of an eye. The intense reaction will lead to severe palpebral oedema, chemosis, and a purulent discharge. While superficial lesions are accompanied by pain, photophobia, and lacrimation, these corneal symptoms may be absent in severe cases because the nerves have been destroyed.

An entirely different reaction occurs with molten metal of relatively low melting point, such as lead, tin, or zinc, which cause less damage. Accidents generally occur when pouring metals into moulds. The metal forms a thin mould over the eye, which can be picked off. Generally the tissue remains undamaged, but occasionally the cornea may be 'dull'. The conjunctiva may be oedematous in the contact area and plaques of encrusted metal may cause superficial burns of the palpebral skin and lid margins, where metal beads have adhered to the eye lashes. Vision is usually unimpaired, although small areas of symblepharon may result.

A burn to the cornea produces irregularity of its thickness and surface, and opacities that give distressing effects upon vision. Contact lenses may restore useful vision in mild cases but corneal grafting may be needed if more severe.

Scalds

Burns by hot fluids frequently affect the lids and face, but the eyes are protected by the blink reflex. Scalds may be caused by ruptures of pipes containing steam or due to splashes of pitch, tar, molten sulphur or boiling oil. Hence, there is usually partial skin loss of the face and lids.

Electrical injuries

Lightning and high tension electrical appliances are the two main causes of electrical injury. An electrical current may generate temperatures of up to 3000 °C on a surface at the point of entry and exit. While tissues are generally bad conductors, nerve tissue conducts extremely well. If the current passes through the head, the hair, eyebrows, and eyelashes will be singed, with superficial burns of the lids, usually associated with marked swelling and conjunctival chemosis. The cornea becomes cloudy due to interstitial opacities and oedema. There may also be iritis, hyphaema, miosis, slow pupil reactions, retinal oedema, papilloedema, retinal detachment, choroidal rupture, chorioretinal atrophy, vitreous opacities, or anterior cortical cataracts (Duke-Elder 1972). The cataracts may have a delayed onset and are, in some cases, transient. A subcapsular cataract in the shape of a fern leaf was reported to have developed in the right eye of a 21-year-old man 6 days after being struck by lightning. The opacity resolved within a few weeks. Another case showed a permanent band-shaped subcapsular cataract and anterior uveitis (Novitskaya and Novitski 1983).

Van Johnson *et al.* (1987) reported cataract formation as a result of electrocution by a high voltage power line which fell on a worker. Diffuse anterior subcapsular cataracts were seen in both eyes 6 weeks after the accident. These progressed to complete subcapsular cataracts and the left eye also developed a diffuse posterior subcapsular cataract. An extracapsular cataract extraction was performed on the left eye.

Figure 5.1 summarizes some of the ocular complications of electrical injuries.

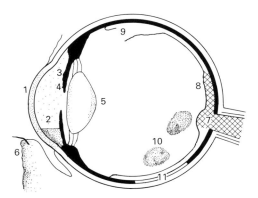

Fig. 5.1 Some of the possible ocular effects of electrical injuries. 1, corneal oedema and interstitial opacities; 2, hyphaema; 3, iritis; 4, miosis; 5, subcapsular cataracts; 6, superficial burns; 7, Papilloedema; 8, retinal oedema; 9, retinal detachment; 10, vitreous opacities; 11, chorioretinal atrophy.

Radiation injuries*

This section examines ocular injuries arising from different radiation sources. First, the electromagnetic spectrum with its radiant energy, both ionizing and non-ionizing, is discussed. While the sun is the principle and natural source of such radiation, there are, of course, man-made sources, such as lasers. We shall also look at ophthalmic instruments in which such sources are used.

Electromagnetic spectrum

The electromagnetic spectrum consists of radiant energy. It comprises a large range of wavelengths, which extend from very short cosmic rays to the much longer Hertzian waves. The major natural source of electromagnetic radiation is the sun. Fortunately, the atmosphere acts as a filter, absorbing a significant amount of the harmful radiations. Ozone and oxygen absorb most of the UV radiation between 10 and 250 nm and water and carbon dioxide absorbs some of the infra-red (IR) radiation. The highest intensity of radiation that penetrates the atmosphere is in the visible range 400–800 nm. Figure 5.2 shows the various wavelengths of the electromagnetic spectrum. At present, the protection provided by the atmosphere and the ocular media against the harmful radiations appears to be adequate. However, there is currently great concern about the thinning of the ozone layer and the resultant health hazards, such as skin cancer.

Damage to the eyes occurs as a result of absorption of harmful radiation, and the effect upon the eye will depend upon the wavelength of the radiation and the photon energy (Lerman 1980a):

1. Long wavelength radiation has low photon energies (< 1 eV) and, when it is absorbed, it will induce rotational and vibrational changes in the molecules. This increase in molecular agitation is generally referred to as a thermal effect.

2. Visible and short wavelength radiations have higher photon energies. The absorption of photon energies from 1 to 4 eV results in changes to the electron energies within the molecule. This excitation of the electrons may be large enough to break some of the chemical bonds and even cause ionization (usually due to absorption of photon energies > 6 eV).

Figure 5.3 illustrates the sites of absorption of the various wavelengths and hence the potential sites of damage. The eye and the skin are particularly sensitive to the non-ionizing radiation normally present in our environment (280–1400 nm). IR radiation does not cause any damage at normal ambient levels, whereas UV radiation can affect both the skin and eye. Most ionizing radiation passes through the eye.

The effect of non-ionizing radiation depends upon the presence of absorbing molecules, known as chromophores. Cells that do not contain chromophores will transmit the wavelengths. Nucleic acids, for example (which are present in the cornea), absorb UV radiation (250–295 nm) but

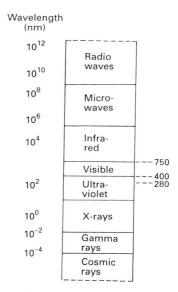

Wavelength (nm)

Fig. 5.2 The electromagnetic spectrum.

---

* This section is mainly summarized from Duke-Elder (1972), Lerman (1980a), Marshall (1985), and Waxler and Hitchins (1986).

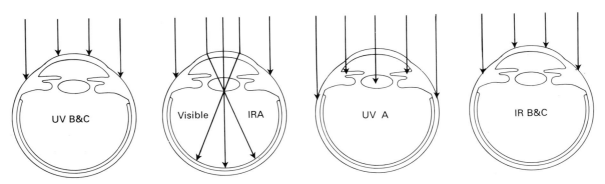

Fig. 5.3 Sites of radiation absorption (reproduced by kind permission of J. Marshall and Butterworth–Heinemann (Oxford) Ltd, 1985).

transmit visible light. Rhodopsin absorbs at 498 nm and haemoglobin absorbs in the UV and visible region (275, 400, and 540–576 nm, respectively) (Lerman 1980a).

The ocular effects of the various wavelengths will now be discussed, and each section will include details on sources, site of absorption, and ocular effects:

(1) ionizing radiation;
(2) non-ionizing radiation:
    (a) ultraviolet radiation;
    (b) visible light;
    (c) infra-red radiation;
    (d) microwave radiation.

Ionizing radiation

SOURCE

Ionizing radiation consists of very short wavelengths (< 0.01 nm) and is caused by the disintegration of atoms. This occurs naturally as cosmic radiation from radioactive isotopes, such as radium, or can be produced by artifical means. These artificial sources can produce X- and gamma-radiation, as well as corpuscular radiation, which includes alpha- and beta-particles, electrons, positrons, protons, and neutrons. People employed in occupations such as radiology, nuclear physics, and uranium mining and engineering, can be at risk from ionizing radiations.

SITE OF ABSORPTION

Most of the ionizing radiation passes through the eye, but a small amount is absorbed and, depending upon the exposure time and concentration, can cause damage to nearly all of the ocular tissues. In general, low penetrating radiations, such as beta-particles, require excessive and repeated exposure for damage, usually cataracts, to occur, whereas high penetrating radiations, such as X- and gamma-radiation and neutrons, require relatively small doses (Duke-Elder 1972).

OCULAR EFFECTS

Many possible changes may occur to ocular tissue when it is exposed to ionizing radiation. The sensitivity of the various ocular tissues will depend upon the miotic activity of the cells, i.e. division and growth, and its ability to repair radiation-induced damage; the fetal eye is far more sensitive to radiation exposure than the adult eye. Of the ocular tissues the conjunctiva, cornea, and lens are most susceptible, as they undergo constant replication and, in the case of the lens, growth throughout life. Merriam and Focht (1962) and Merriam *et al.* (1972) have listed the relative sensitivity of the ocular tissues in decreasing order: (i) lens; (ii) conjunctiva; (iii) cornea; (iv) vitreous; (v) iris and uveal tract; (vi) sclera; and (vii) retina.

The ionizing radiation may have a direct or an indirect effect upon the tissues. A direct action upon the cells can result in the development of abnormalities, or in cell death. Indirect damage can occur as a result of damage of the blood vessels, leading to a reduced blood supply to the tissues.

The most common effect of radiation exposure is the formation of cataracts, because the lens contains the ocular tissues that are most sensitive to this type of radiation. The lenticular changes are similar regardless of the type of radiation—fine dot-like subcapsular opacities in the anterior cortex and granular and vacuolar subcapsular opacities at the posterior pole of the lens. These may progress to involve the peripheral portions of the posterior cortex (Palva and Palkama 1978; Hayes and Fisher 1979). It may take several years for the cataracts to develop after exposure to the radiation. The latent period and the severity of lens damage depends on:

1. *Radiation dose.* Duration and concentration: single or multiple exposure. A single dose of 250 rad appears to be the threshold level above which the radiation is capable of inducing cataracts in humans. (Rad is defined as the absorbed dose of radiation when 1 g of material absorbs 100 ergs of energy; 1 rad = 10^{-2} J kg^{-1}.) However, dose-splitting can increase the threshold to 550 rad if the doses are spread over 3 months (Merriam and Focht 1957).

2. *Type of radiation.* Low or high penetration.

3. *Age of person.* The younger the person the shorter the latent period and the greater the lens damage.

When a patient is undergoing radiation treatment for ocular tumours, such as retinoblastoma, there is the risk of unwanted side-effects, e.g. cataract formation. If the eyelids are being irradiated because of the presence of a basal cell carcinoma, the eye should be protected by a lead contact lens. Unfortunately, the loss of lashes, pigmentary changes to the skin, and 'dry eye' due to atrophy of the accessory lacrimal glands, are not easy to prevent.

Non-ionizing radiation

Ultraviolet radiation
SOURCE
Table 5.4 shows the range of wavelengths in the UV region and their sources. UV radiation ranges from 200 to 400 nm and can be subdivided into three groups: (i) UV-A, 315–400 nm; (ii) UV-B, 280–315 nm; and (iii) UV-C, 200–280 nm. The most common sources of UV radiation,

Table 5.4 Ultraviolet radiation and the eye (courtesy of J. Marshall and Butterworth–Heinemann (Oxford) Ltd 1985)

Spectral domain		Wavelength (nm)	Sources	Site of ocular damage
Biological	Physical			
UV-C	Far UV	200–280	Sunlight Lamps—arc, germicidal mercury Excimer laser	Corneal epithelium resulting in photokeratitis, corneal opacity
UV-B	Far UV	280–315	Sunlight Sunlamps Welding arc Excimer laser	Corneal epithelium Resulting in photokeratitis, corneal opacity
		295–315		Lens epithelium and nucleus Resulting in cataract
UV-A	Near UV	315–400	Sunlight UV-A sunlamp Sunbeds Excimer laser	Lens epithelium and nucleus Resulting in cataract

apart from sunlight, are germicidal lamps, high pressure mercury arc lamps, fluorescent lamps, and welding arcs. Of particular concern is the increasing use of sunlamps and sunbeds, which are sources of UV-A and UV-B.

SITE OF ABSORPTION
The corneal epithelium and conjunctiva absorb the wavelengths between 200 and 315 nm (UV-C and UV-B) and the lens nucleus and epithelium absorbs the wavelengths between 295 and 400 nm (i.e. UV-A and part UV-B; see Fig. 5.3). With age, the filtering effect of the crystalline lens increases as a result of the increase in concentration of chromophores, which absorb the radiation. Therefore, most of the UV radiation is absorbed by the cornea, and some by the crystalline lens, and photo-chemical damage results.

OCULAR EFFECTS
UV radiation can act upon the eye by two mechanisms: (i) direct: radiation is absorbed by chromophores within the tissue; and (ii) indirect: radiation is absorbed by photosensitizing drugs or other compounds.

DIRECT EFFECTS OF UV RADIATION
Cornea—photokeratitis
UV-B and UV-C are absorbed by the corneal epithelium, which results in a reduction of the cell division in mild cases or, in severe cases, in

complete death of the epithelial cells and loss of injured cells. Corneal ulceration may occur in extreme cases (English 1973). The accumulation of damaged and exfoliated cells on the surface of the cornea can act as an effective filter to limit the total exposure dose and filter specific wavelengths of UV radiation.

Unfortunately, the eye cannot built up resistance to UV radiation, like the skin does; exposure has an accumulative effect in a 24-hour period. So, while a single exposure may not be harmful, if repeated the accumulative effect may be above threshold and result in epithelial damage (English 1973; Cullen 1980).

The maximum efficiency for experimental photokeratitis is seen to occur at 288–290 nm, with a small peak at 254–260 nm (Bachem 1956; Pitts and Tredici 1971). These peaks correspond to the presence of the absorbing chromophores in the cornea (nucleic acids at 260 nm and tyrosine and tryptophan at 275–290 nm).

Following exposure to UV radiation, there is a latent period of 6–12 h before any symptoms are noticed. This period varies inversely with the dose of UV radiation exposure. The symptoms experienced are:

(1) a sensation of sand in the eyes, due to congestion of the conjunctival and episcleral blood vessels;
(2) lacrimation;
(3) photophobia;
(4) chemosis;
(5) blepharospasm;
(6) erythema (redness) of the lids.

The condition is generally self-limiting and almost all the discomfort disappears within 48 h due to the repair mechanisms of the corneal epithelium. Photokeratitis is common amongst welders, when the condition is referred to as 'arc eye' or 'welder's flash'.

The latent period appears to be due to a marked decrease in corneal sensitivity. A study by Millodot and Earlam (1984) found that after exposure to UV radiation from an electric arc welder the corneal sensitivity decreased. The sensation of sand and pain in the eyes is experienced as the corneal sensitivity is restored (Fig. 5.4).

Therapy consists of instillation of lubricating ointment and decongestant drops. A local/topical anaesthetic can be given and the eye can be patched if pain is severe and blepharospasm is present.

Although the primary short-term effect of acute exposures of UV radiation to the cornea is photokeratitis, damage to the corneal endothelium may also occur (Cullen *et al.* 1984). It also appears that chronic UV radiation exposure contributes to increased endothelial polymegethism seen with age (Good and Schoessler 1988).

Pingecula, pterygium, and band-shaped keratopathy

Long-term chronic exposure to UV radiation is thought to be partly responsible for other conditions, namely pingeculae pterygia, and band—shaped keratopathies. A significantly high incidence of pingeculae and pterygia is found amongst outdoor workers, such as fishermen and welders,

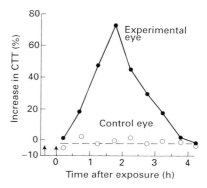

Fig. 5.4 Corneal sensitivity after absorption of UV radiation. (The arrows indicate UV exposure; CTT, corneal touch threshold (reproduced by kind permission of Millodot, M., Earlam, R.A. and publishers S. Karger AG 1984.)

who are exposed to UV radiation (Klintworth 1972; Norm 1982, Karai and Horiguchi 1984; Moran and Hollows 1984; Mackenzie *et al.* 1992).

A nodular band-shaped keratopathy has been noted in people who live in areas of the world with high levels of UV. White or cream opacities occur between the epithelium and Bowman's membrane in the palperal fissure (Rodger 1973). Anderson and Fuglsang (1976) also reported similar degenerative changes of the cornea associated with UV exposure.

Cataracts

The crystalline lens epithelium and nucleus absorb wavelengths between 295 and 400 nm, i.e. part of UV-B and UV-A. As only the shorter wave lengths are filtered out by the cornea, the lens is constantly exposed to the longer wavelengths (between 295 and 400 nm) throughout life. It has been shown that these wavelengths are responsible for generating fluorescent compounds, and for the protein cross-linking associated with lens ageing and cataract formation. A young lens will transmit approximately 90 per cent of incident light > 400 nm but with age the amount of short-wave radiation transmitted is reduced, particularly in the region of 300–400 nm (Lerman 1980*a*; Lerman 1983).

Chronic cumulative photochemical damage results in increased absorption of UV radiation and some visible light due to photochemically generated chromophores. The chromophores increase in concentration and number with age and are responsible for the increased yellow colour of the lens nucleus, and hence enable the lens to act as an effective filter, protecting the retina from cumulative photochemical damage by the second to third decade (Weale 1983; Zigman 1983).

Lerman (1980*b*) reported that 'senile' cataracts have occurred at an earlier age (40–50 years) in workers exposed to industrial sources of UV-A, e.g. printing works, dentistry, and medicine. So is there any evidence to suggest that exposure to UV radiation is responsible for cataract formation?

Many papers now suggest that UV radiation is a causative factor in cataract formation. Animal studies have shown that cataracts can be induced by UV radiation. One study found that high doses were required in the region between 295 and 320 nm to produce cataracts (Bachem 1956), whilst another found that long-term exposure can also produce cataracts, usually anterior subcapsular cataracts (Zigman and Vaughn 1974). Other studies have established threshold levels of exposure for near UV radiation. However, permanent lens changes were not induced until the radiant exposure levels reached twice the threshold value (Pitts 1978). Epidemiological studies are also inconclusive. Some have shown that in areas of high levels of sunlight and UV radiation there is a higher incidence of cataracts (Hiller *et al.* 1977; Hollows and Moran 1981; Zigman 1983), whilst one reported a lower incidence (Crabbe 1983). The different results in these studies may well be due to such factors as general health and diet, that were not taken into account (Minassian *et al.* 1984).

It has also been suggested that the brown (brunescent) cataract that occurs in the nucleus of the older lens results from exposure to sunlight. However, this has not yet been proven and there are major arguments against the hypothesis (Harding and Dilley 1976).

To summarize, although the evidence is not entirely conclusive as to the relationship between UV radiation and cataracts, it would seem sensible to assume from all the research so far that a causal relationship is possible (Pitts 1981).

A summary of the possible anterior segment complications of UV radiation are shown in Figure 5.5.

Vitreous shrinkage
The vitreous is normally protected from damage by the cornea and lens, which filter wavelengths up to 400 nm. However, if the eye is aphakic the vitreous has no protection against wave lengths > 295 nm. The vitreous gel possesses UV-absorbing chromophores and there is experimental evidence that damage, such as vitreous shrinkage and denaturation of the collagen network, can occur (Balazs *et al.* 1959).

Retina
As stated above, the retina is generally protected from UV radiation by the cornea and lens, but damage can occur to: (i) aphakes who lack the filtering effect of the lens; and (ii) fishermen and sailors or employees in industries where UV polymerization is employed.

Aphakes are prone to cystoid macula oedema. This is now thought to be due to absorption of the wavelengths > 295 nm. A study by Kraff *et al.* (1985) reported that patients who had been given UV-absorbing intra-ocular lenses after cataract extraction had a lower incidence of cystoid macula oedema than those who did not receive absorbing implants. However, this report did not describe the absorption characteristics of the eye, intra-ocular lenses, and spectacles. Wittenberg (1986) makes the point that, until Kraff *et al.*'s study, there were no reports of apparent retinal damage in people who had been aphakic from an early age. Therefore, the association between retinal damage and UV radiation due to sunlight is uncertain.

The aphakic eye is also at risk from retinal detachments due to vitreous shrinkage and denaturation of the collagen network. Ageing is known to cause a loss of rod and cone cells, and it has been suggested that this is due to a potential cumulative action of light, i.e. a phototoxic effect, which is cumulative in the normal ageing process. As studies suggest that UV and short-wave visible radiation (320–450 nm) are significant factors in retinal photochemical damage, it is advisable to provide protection, especially for aphakics, by giving UV-absorbing spectacle lenses or intra-ocular lenses.

INDIRECT EFFECTS OF UV RADIATION
There are reports that UV radiation can be indirectly absorbed by photo-sensitizing drugs and cause damage to the crystalline lens and retina (Lerman *et al.* 1980; Boukes *et al.* 1985; Woo 1985). A treatment for psoriasis, known as PUVA therapy, consists of the ingestion of a psoralen compound (e.g. 8-methoxypsoralens (8-MOP) or methoxalen) followed by exposure to UV-A radiation. Ocular protection must be provided as the UV-A radiation causes binding of the psoralen compound to lens and retinal proteins in aphakic individuals. This protection must be provided for at least 12–24h after ingestion, i.e. until there is no psoralen compound

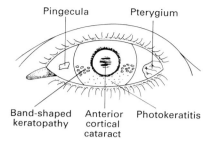

Fig. 5.5 Some of the possible effects of UV radiation on the anterior segment of the eye.

Table 5.5 Visible radiation and the eye (courtesy of J. Marshall and Butterworth–Heinemann (Oxford) Ltd 1985)

Visible wave length (nm)	Sources	Site of ocular damage
400–780	Sunlight Lamps—incandescent fluorescent, arc Lasers—argon, krypton	Retinal piment epithelium, haemoglobin, macular pigment, photoreceptors Resulting in visual loss, colour vision problems, accelerated ageing

remaining in the lens (Boukes *et al.* 1985). The opacities occur in the anterior and posterior cortical layers; some are punctate and others are wedge-shaped. It is believed that the opacification is mainly due to binding of tryptophan and lens proteins, which remain in the lens (Lerman *et al.* 1980).

Visible light
SOURCES AND SITE OF ABSORPTION
Table 5.5 shows the sources and site of absorption of visible light. The range of visible radiation is from 400–780 nm, most of which reaches the retina.

OCULAR EFFECTS
Visible light may cause damage by thermal photocoagulation. Retinal burns may occur when high intensities of light are focused on the retina. The severity of the damage will depend upon the intensity of the source. Non-thermal damage can occur with long-term exposure to ambient light levels with intensities well below that required to cause thermal damage.

Experimental animal studies have shown that retinal damage can occur at relatively low levels of visible radiation energy and, hence, there is concern that such exposure may be responsible for retinal degeneration in humans (Noell *et al.* 1966; Kuwabara and Gorn 1968; O'Steen *et al.* 1972; Lanum 1978; Ham *et al.* 1982). The long-term exposure to low levels of visible and UV radiation has been shown to cause damage to the photoreceptors, especially the cones, and to the retinal pigment epithelium (Heriot 1985; Marshall 1985; Mainster 1987; Young 1988). It appears that the overloading of the photopigments results in a chain of metabolic events, which can lead to reversible or irreversible damage to the photoreceptors. Whether the damage to the retinal pigment epithelium occurs before or at the same time as the damage to the photoreceptors, remains an open question.

The following degenerative changes are believed to occur to the rods and cones (Kuwabara and Gorn 1968):

1. Vacuole formation of the outer tip of the photoreceptor.
2. The outer segment loses its lamellar structure and becomes tortuous and swollen.
3. The outer segment breaks off from the inner segment.
4. The outer segments are phagocytosed by retinal pigment epithelium.
5. Photoreceptors disappear but remaining layers are intact.

The cones appear to be more sensitive to photopic damage than the rods (Marshall *et al.* 1972; Sykes *et al.* 1981) and especially sensitive to the blue region of visible light and UV (Harwerth and Sperling 1971). Marshall (1985) has suggested that the difference in sensitivity between the rods and cones is not due to a difference in threshold for damage, but rather to different capacities for repair. There has been concern about the output of various light sources and their potential hazards (Sliney and Wolbarsht 1980). Artificial illumination levels generally vary between 200–500 lm/m^2. These levels are below levels of irradiance producing retinal photopathology in primates and man. However, the trend for higher lighting levels should be approached with caution in view of the photic damage that may be incurred at these high levels (Lerman 1987).

Infra-red radiation
SOURCES AND SITE OF ABSORPTION
The range of infra-red wavelengths lies between 780 and 10 000 nm (Table 5.6). It can be subdivided into three groups: (i) IR-A, 780–1400 nm; IR-B, 1400–3000 nm; IR-C, 3000–10 000 nm. Wavelengths of 3000 nm and longer do not usually reach our environment because they are absorbed by the atmosphere. The most common sources of IR radiation are sunlight, arc lamps, electric fires, and steel and glass furnaces.

Table 5.6 Infra-red radiation and the eye (courtesy of J. Marshall and Butterworth–Heinemann (Oxford) Ltd 1985)

Spectral domain		Wave length (nm)	Sources	Site of ocular damage
Biological	Physical			
IR-A	Near IR	780–1,400	Sunlight, furnaces, arc lamp, electric fires, Neodymium YAG laser	Pigment epithelium of retina, iris, lens Resulting in visual loss and cataract
IR-B	Far IR	1,400–3,000	Sunlight, furnaces, Erbium laser	Corneal and lens epithelium Resulting in corneal opacity, aqueous flare and cataract
IR-C	Far IR	3,000–10,000	Furnaces, carbon dioxide laser	Corneal epithelium Resulting in corneal opacity

IR radiation, when absorbed, leads to rotational and vibrational changes, which result in a thermal effect on the tissue. The major sites of absorption are shown in Figure 5.3. The cornea absorbs wave lengths > 3000 nm, i.e. IR-C; the crystalline lens absorbs wavelengths < 3000 nm, i.e. IR-A and IR-B; and the retina absorbs wave lengths < 1400 nm, i.e. IR-A. There is some absorption in all the ocular tissues, but the absorption by the crystalline lens and retina are of greatest concern.

OCULAR EFFECTS
The damage that occurs to the eye after absorption of IR radiation is due to thermal effects.

Cornea
Absorption by the cornea of IR-C results in opacification, especially of the stroma, due to thermal photocoagulation of the corneal proteins.

Crystalline lens
Cataracts generally occur to workers who are exposed to intense heat for many years, i.e. steelworkers and glass blowers. The opacification occurs in the cortex of the crystalline lens. It is often associated with lamellar splitting and exfoliation of the anterior lens capsule. This damage results from both direct and indirect absorption of IR radiation. Indirect absorption by the pigment epithelium of the iris results in a heat transfer to the underlying lens. This may lead to anterior subcapsular opacities (Langely *et al.* 1960; Pitts and Cullen 1981). Direct absorption at the posterior pole of the lens where radiation from a large source is focused, may induce posterior cortical or subcapsular cataracts (Goldman 1935; Edbrooke and Edwards 1967).

Retina
Retinal burns have been reported after exposure to IR radiations (750–1400 nm) in a variety of conditions, such as solar retinopathy (Agarwal and Malik 1959; Tso and La Piana 1975), eclipse blindness (Penner and McNair 1966), exposure to high intensity light sources such as xenon lamps, MIG (metal-arc inertgas) welders (Brittain 1988) and exposure to IR lasers. The IR radiation is focused on the retina and will be absorbed by the melanin pigment granules in the pigment epithelium and underlying choroid. This results in a thermal reaction and inflammatory response involving the neural retina.

Microwave radiation

SOURCES
Microwave radiation consists of wavelengths ranging from 1 mm to 30 cm, with frequencies ranging from 10^9 Hz up to 3×10^{11} Hz. There has been a rapid increase in the use of microwave radiations, for example, in microwave ovens, FM radio, television, and radar.

SITE OF ABSORPTION
The direct effect of microwave radiation is due to an increase in temperature of the tissue. The absorption depends on:

(1) type of tissue;
(2) wavelength;
(3) frequency.

Tissue
Water-based tissue absorbs much more energy than fat or bone, which microwaves can penetrate with little loss of energy. Tissues with higher amounts of water and greater conductivity, such as muscle tissue, will absorb the microwave energy, which results in a temperature rise. Conduction and convection of the heat will diminish the temperature differences induced by the absorption of the microwave radiation.

The relative avascularity of the intra-ocular cavity will result in a temperature increase within the eye. This is markedly higher than in other, well-vascularized tissues absorbing an equivalent amount of radiation. The crystalline lens is avascular and hence its inability to dissipate heat, is particularly prone to thermal damage from microwave radiation. From experimental animal studies the dose required to produce a cataract is believed to be 100–150 mW/cm² (Richardson *et al.* 1951; Daily *et al.* 1952; Williams *et al.* 1955).

Wavelength
The degree of penetration of microwave radiation is directly related to the wavelength. The thermal effects of the longer wavelengths are more penetrating. For example, a 12 cm microwave will penetrate about 1 cm into the eye, compared to a 1 mm penetration by a 3 cm wave. The temperature gradients created by different wavelengths is shown in Figure 5.6 (Richardson *et al.* 1951). The maximum temperature rise occurs in the posterior cortex of the lens when exposed to 12 cm microwaves, whereas the maximum temperature rise occurs in the cornea for 3 cm microwaves.

Frequency
There is a relationship between the microwave frequency and the amount of absorption. The amount absorbed at the surface of exposed tissues increases with increasing microwave frequency (Schwan and Piersal 1954).

OCULAR EFFECTS
Ocular effects of microwaves can only be assessed by experimental or clinical means. The experimental production of anterior and posterior subcapsular cataracts in animals at relatively high intensities (> 100 mW/cm²) has been documented by several researchers (Daily *et al.* 1952; Van Ummerson and Cogan 1965; Stewart-DeHann *et al.* 1985). However, it is believed by some that lower levels of microwave exposure can also induce cataracts if there are repeated exposures to subthreshold doses. It appears that cell membrane damage is responsible for cataract formation (Lipman *et al.* 1988).

The only available human data are from retrospective population surveys comparing microwave workers with controls matched for age and sex. So far all population surveys have failed to show a correlation between occupational exposure and cataract formation. One of the largest surveys was carried out by Appleton *et al.* (1975) of 2343 military personnel. They

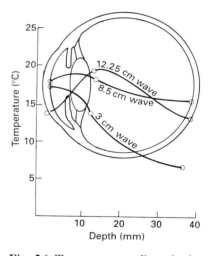

Fig. 5.6 Temperature gradients in the exposed eye to 12.25, 8.5, and 3 cm pulsed microwaves (from Richardson *et al.* 1951, Archives of Ophthalmology, 45:382–386, copyright, 1951, American Medical Association).

concluded that there was no difference in the incidence of lens opacities between the control group and experimental subjects, and that lens damage due to microwave radiation from military equipment had not occurred. These findings suggested that the existing safety level of 10 mW/cm² is adequate. (For a review of the studies, see Lipman *et al.* 1988.)

Instruments using specific man-made sources of radiation
Lasers
SOURCES

The use of laser technology has increased greatly in recent years and lasers have many applications in engineering, science, medicine, and the defence industry. A laser beam is a monochromatic, coherent, parallel, very high energy beam. It is produced by the excitation of atoms to a higher than usual energy state by the input of radiant energy, which causes the emission of light as the atoms return to their original energy state. Many substances can be used as a laser source, e.g. ruby, argon, carbon dioxide, or YAG (yttrium–aluminium–garnet). 'Laser' is an acronym for 'Light Amplification by Stimulated Emission of Radiation'. Lasers have been produced to emit at many monochromatic wavelengths ranging from far UV (< 300 nm) to far IR (> 1400 nm).

Different types of exposure can be produced from a laser depending upon the mode of operation (Lerman 1980*a*; Mainster *et al.* 1983*b*):

1. *Continuous wave mode.* In which the exposure time can vary from a few milliseconds to minutes.
2. *Long pulsed mode.* In which the exposure time ranges from 100 μs to 2 ms.
3. *Q-switched mode.* In which the exposure time is less than 100 ns (1 ns = 10^{-9} s).
4. *Mode-locked.* In which the time exposure may vary from 20–40 ps pulses (1 ps = 10^{-12} s).

The Q-switched mode and mode-locked methods of operation allow high peaked power to be produced by compressing the laser output in time.

There are four important radiometric terms in medical laser applications: (i) energy measured in joules (J); (ii) power measured in watts (W); (iii) radiant energy density measured in joules per cm² (J/cm²); and (iv) irradiance measured in watts per cm² (W/cm²). (1 joule = 1 watt × 1 second). The laser output is quantified in joules or watts and its effect upon the tissue is determined by the spot size, which will determine the energy density or irradiance. The power of a continuous beam laser, such as an argon laser, is measured in watts, while pulsed lasers (e.g. neodymium (Nd): YAG) provide a reading of energy per pulse in joules.

Continuous wave laser systems, such as argon and krypton lasers, focus light energy on an area of tissue to cause a temperature rise, which in turn causes coagulation of the tissue. The temperature rise depends on the spot size, amount of energy, and wavelength. The wavelength determines the efficiency with which the light source is absorbed and converted into heat by the pigment of the tissues (Mainster *et al.* 1970, 1983*a*). An excessive temperature rise can cause an explosion and haemorrhage in the tissue. Only a 10 °C rise in temperature is required for retinal

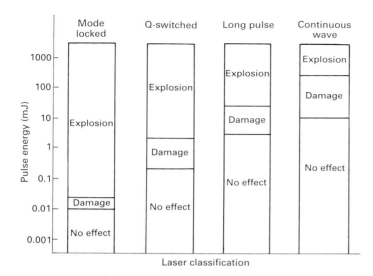

Fig. 5.7 Pulse energy required to produce retinal damage or haemorrhage for laser exposures of different durations (after Mainster *et al.* 1983, published courtesy of *Ophthalmology*).

photocoagulation. Short pulse lasers, such as Nd:YAG, will disrupt transparent tissue, and hence are known as photodisruptors. They are generally used for the relatively transparent anterior portion of the eye.

There are various mechanisms whereby the short pulse laser systems disrupt the transparent membranes (Mainster *et al.* 1983*b*):

1. The high irradiance (power/area) disintegrates tissues by removing electrons from atoms (i.e. ionizing them) and creating a 'plasma', which is a gaseous state consisting of electrons and ions.
2. The rapid outwards expansion of the plasma creates shock and acoustic waves, which mechanically disrupt adjacent tissue.
3. Latent stress in the membrane causes further disruption.
4. A specific photochemical reaction has been reported with UV lasers, which results in the ablation of corneal tissues without thermal damage to the adjacent structures (Trokel *et al.* 1983).

Figure 5.7 shows the pulse energy required to produce retinal damage for laser exposures of different durations (Mainster *et al.* 1983*b*). It can be seen that mode-locked exposures are potentially more hazardous than Q-switched, and that short pulses can produce retinal damage with less energy (or irradiance) than the longer pulse. The margin between retinal damage and explosion is also much lower for short pulse than for continuous wave.

Site of absorption
The site of absorption depends upon the wavelength being emitted by the laser. Radiation from lasers emitting in the UV region will be absorbed by the cornea and crystalline lens. Visible and IR lasers will cause problems, not necessarily because of their power but due to the fact that the collimated beam will be focused on to the retina.

OCULAR EFFECTS

UV lasers emitting radiation < 300 nm can be absorbed by the cornea and, as described, will cause damage to the corneal epithelium. Lasers emitting UV from 300–400 nm can cause cataracts because the radiation is absorbed by the crystalline lens. UV-emitting lasers can therefore cause damage to the cornea and crystalline lens, if they are exposed for a sufficient time and at power densities above threshold level. As a result of this, the Excimer laser is now being used, particularly for corneal surgery, as the depth of incision can be accurately controlled by the photons that break the molecular bonds when absorbed. This has the advantage that the adjacent tissue does not suffer from thermal damage. Marshall *et al.* (1986) found that the wavelength of 193 nm was optimal for corneal surgery. The Excimer laser was initially used in the printing and electronics industries, where its properties allowed submicron patterns to be etched into the surface of materials without damaging the adjacent non-irradiated areas. A study by Trokel *et al.* (1983) shows that $1 J/cm^2$ ablates corneal tissue to a depth of 1 μm.

The wavelengths of visible and IR lasers are focused on to the retina, where they cause damage:

1. *Thermal injury*. Absorption by the melanin, the pigment epithelium, and choroid.
2. *Photochemical damage*. Especially in the blue region of the visible spectrum, which is absorbed by the inner retinal layers.
3. *Shock waves*. These are produced by the Q-switched high intensity beams, which cause disruption of the internal cellular structure.

The type and degree of retinal damage caused by a laser will depend upon (Ham *et al.* 1970):

(1) the power density of the laser (W/cm^2);
(2) time of exposure;
(3) the wavelength and transmission through the ocular media;
(4) the size of image upon the retina;
(5) the blink reflex;
(6) the degree of retinal and choroidal pigmentation.

Industrial ocular laser burns have been reported by Boldrey *et al.* (1981). The damage ranged from minor retinal burns to extensive areas of damage with retinal oedema and vitreous haemorrhages. A variety of lasers were involved, including Nd:YAG, argon, krypton, and rhodamine dye. The haemorrhages and oedema subsided during the weeks following the injury and, with the exception of one case, the final visual acuity was 6/6, although a paracentral scotoma was usually present. In all but one case eye protection was not being worn; in the case where eye protection was being worn, it was not fitted correctly and the spectacles slipped as the worker bent over the laser, the beam being reflected from a piece of test paper into his left eye. There are other reports of ocular injury from lasers where the visual outcome was not as good. Many of the cases resulted in a markedly reduced final vision, one case being due to a macula hole (Jacobson and McLean 1965; Rathkey 1965; Zweng 1967; Curtin and Boyden 1968; Armstrong 1970; Henkes and Zuidema 1975).

Ophthalmic instruments

There is concern that radiation from ophthalmic instruments may cause damage to the eye being examined, especially the retina. The proceedings of a symposium on intense light hazards in ophthalmic diagnosis and treatment (Calkins *et al.* 1980) have shown that various ophthalmic instruments are capable of causing damage to the retina. Estimates were made of the critical exposure time for the retina with the indirect ophthalmoscope, slit lamp, operating microscope, and overhead surgical lamp. The retinal irradiance of the instruments was calculated for a person with clear ocular media and a dilated pupil. This was correlated with the recommended maximum permissible exposure (MPE) time based on the ANSI Z-136 guidelines for laser safety to provide a safe viewing time for the various instruments (Table 5.7). The 'safe time' indicates how long exposure at the particular level of retinal irradiance must be maintained before the ANSI laser safety guidelines are exceeded ($2.92 \, J/cm^2$). However, these studies did not take into account the spectral power distribution of the light sources.

OPHTHALMOSCOPES

Indirect ophthalmoscopes can produce levels of retinal irradiance up to five times greater than that produced by a direct ophthalmoscope. There are obviously differences between the types of ophthalmoscopes, for example the Keeler Indirect produces nearly 3.6 times more irradiance than the

Table 5.7 Safe viewing time for various ophthalmic instruments (reprinted with permission of Vision Research, vol. 20, Calkins et al., Potential hazards from specific ophthalmic devices. Copyright 1980, Pergamon Press plc).

Instrument	Average retinal irradiance (mW/cm^2)	Safe time(s)*
Direct ophthalmoscope (A.O. Giantscope: Welch Allyn)	29.0	–
Indirect ophthalmoscopes (Binocular-AO and Frigi-Xonix)	68.6 6.5 V 125.0 7.8–8.4 V	42 23
Slit lamp (Haag Streit)	140.0 5 V 217.0 6 V 358.0 7.5 V	21 13 8
Operating microscope emmetrope and myopes	100.0–970	29–1.8
aphakic	59.0–590	49–3.7

* Safe time is defined as the time required to reach an integrated retinal irradiance of $2.92 \, J/cm^2$.

American Optical at maximum voltage setting (Kossel *et al.* 1983). The power of the condensing lens also affects the retinal irradiance, which increases as the power of the condensing lens decreases. A 14 D lens can give 81 per cent more retinal irradiance than a 20 D lens (Calkins *et al.* 1980).

Therefore, an indirect ophthalmoscope is considered to be unsafe, when compared with the laser safety standard, after 23 s exposure in a normal patient with clear media and dilated pupils. The time taken for fundus examination should not, therefore, be prolonged unnecessarily.

The light sources in ophthalmoscopes are usually an incandescent bulb (tungsten halogen) and are composed of one-third visible and UV radiation, and two-thirds IR radiation. It has therefore been suggested that an IR filter should be incorporated in all ophthalmoscopes to avoid thermal damage from extensive viewing (Lerman 1985). The higher the voltage at which the bulbs are operated, the greater the amount of UV radiation emitted. As UV-A and blue light can cause damage to the retina, especially in aphakes whose natural filter has been removed, it has been suggested that a cut-off filter at 450 nm should also be incorporated (Kossol *et al.* 1983; Cullen and Chou 1984).

A recent survey by James *et al.* (1988) has investigated the light hazard of hand-held direct ophthalmoscopes. Studying the spectral irradiance of ophthalmoscopes at maximum output, James *et al.* found that the levels of UV and IR radiation are not hazardous, although they may be potentially harmful to certain groups of patients, such as aphakes. They therefore recommended the use of UV- and IR-blocking filters. For most ophthalmoscopes the safe time was found to be in excess of 1 h.

Slit lamps
Slit lamp examination of the retina produces up to three times more irradiance than indirect ophthalmoscopy. The level of irradiance obviously depends upon the lamp voltage and can range from 140 mW/cm^2 to 358 mW/cm^2 for a 5 and 7.5 V lamp, respectively (Calkins *et al.* 1980). The safe durations for retinal examination are also shorter than for indirect ophthalmoscopy, being as little as 8 s. It has therefore, been suggested that medium voltage settings should be used and that short examination times of 10 s should be employed. This applies particularly to the examination of patients with macular or retinal degenerations.

Operating microscopes
These can produce up to ten times more retinal irradiance than indirect ophthalmoscopes, i.e. up to 970 mW/cm^2. The retinal irradiance, and hence safe times, are seen to vary with the patient's refractive error. The safe time varies from 1.8 to 49 s, which is still relatively short when considering the time taken during operation procedures, (Calkins *et al.* 1980). It has therefore been suggested that corneal occluders should be used during prolonged procedures with operating microscopes. Although microscopes do not produce much UV radiation it is still advisable to incorporate a pale yellow filter to absorb blue light and UV-A. Care should be taken in certain conditions, such as retinitis pigmentosa, when light exposure may accelerate the disease.

Light sources such as the surgical illuminating lid speculum provide a safe retinal irradiance (Calkins *et al.* 1980). It may provide 900 times less retinal irradiance than conventional operating microscopes.

To summarize:

1. Use IR filters to absorb wavelengths longer than 700 nm.
2. Absorb wavelengths below 450 nm to eliminate blue light and UV-A. This will improve image quality by reducing the light scattering and chromatic aberration.
3. Use the minimum amount of light and time necessary for examination.
4. In some cases corneal occluders can be used to prevent unnecessary exposure from operating microscopes.

It is interesting to note that scanning laser ophthalmoscopes have been designed in which the light intensities required for illumination of the retina are considerably less than in conventional instruments (Mainster *et al.* 1982; Plesch *et al.* 1987). In the system described by Mainster *et al.* 1982 the light level was less than $70\,\mu W/cm^2$ compared with $100\,000$ $\mu W/cm^2$ for direct ophthalmoscopes. This means that it is possible to view the retina through an undilated pupil. The examination will be more comfortable for the patient compared with indirect ophthalmoscopy. A laser that emits IR light can also be used to view the retina, and this provides a very comfortable method of examination for the patient who is unaware of the light (Webb *et al.* 1987).

Summary

Chapters 4 and 5 have discussed the various ocular injuries that may occur due to mechanical and non-mechanical hazards. The urgency of attention has been outlined by Fox (1973; Table 5.8). The most urgent

Table 5.8 Urgency for treatment of traumatic ocular injuries (from Fox, S.L. 1973) *Industrial and occupational ophthalmology*. Courtesy of Charles C. Thomas, Springfield, Illinois.)

Group1: True emergencies	Group 2: Urgent conditions	Group 3: Less urgent conditions
Institute therapy immediately for: Chemical burns to the cornea	Penetrating injuries of the globe (cornea or sclera)	Corneal rust deposit
	Corneal erosion, ulcer or abrasion	Fractures about the orbit
	Corneal foreign body	Lacerations of the conjunctiva
	Eyelid laceration	Subluxations of the lens
	Hyphema	
	Acute vitreous haemorrhage	
	Acut retinal tear/detachment	
	Thermal and radiant burns	

condition is that of a chemical burn, which requires immediate action: the eye should be irrigated as soon as possible. Other ocular injuries are listed according to the degree of urgency of the condition.

References

Agarwal, L.P. and Malik, S.R.K. (1959). Solar retinitis. *Br. J. Ophthalmol.*, **53**, 366–70.

Anderson, J. and Fuglsang, (1976). Droplet degeneration of the cornea in the North Cameroon. Prevalence and clinical appearances. *Br. J. Ophthalmol.*, **60**, 256–62.

Appleton, B., Hirsch, S., Kinion, R.O., Soles, M., McCrossan, G.C., and Neidlinger, R.M. (1975). Microwave lens effect in humans II—Results of 5 year survey. *Arch. Ophthalmol.*, **93**, 257–8.

Armstrong, C.E. (1970). Eye injuries in the modern radiation environment. *J. Am. Optom. Assoc.*, **41**, 55–62.

Bachem, A. (1956). Ophthalmic ultra-violet action spectra. *Am. J. Ophthalmol.*, **41**, 969–74.

Balazs, E.A., Laurent, T.C., Howe, F.C., and Varga, L. (1959). Irradiation of mucopolysaccharides with ultraviolet light and electrons. *Radiant. Res.*, **11**, 149–64.

Boldrey, E.E., Little, H.L., Flocks, M., and Vassiliadis, A. (1981). Retinal injury due to industrial laser burns. *Ophthalmology*, **88**, 101–7.

Boukes, R.J., Van Balen, A. Th M., and Bruynzeel, D.P. (1985). A retrospective study of ocular findings in patients treated with PUVA. *Doc. Ophthalmol.*, **59**, 11–19.

Brittain, G.P.H. (1988). Retinal burns caused by exposure to MIG welding arcs: report of two cases. *Br. J. Ophthalmol.*, **72**, 570–5.

Brown, S.I., Akiya, S., and Weller, C.A. (1969). Prevention of ulcers of the cornea: preliminary studies with collagenase inhibitors. *Arch. Ophthalmol.*, **82**, 95–7.

Brown, S.I., Tragakis, M.P., and Pearce, D.B. (1972). Treatment of alkali burned cornea. *Am. J. Ophthalmol.*, **74**, 316–20.

Calkins, J.L., Hochheimer, B.F., and D'Anna, S.A. (1980). Potential hazards from specific ophthalmic devices. *Vis. Res.*, **20**, 1039–53.

Crabbe, M.J.C. (1983). Low incidence of cataract in Hawaii despite high exposure to sunlight. *Lancet*, **1**, 649.

Cullen, A.P. (1980). Additive effects of ultraviolet radiation. *Am. J. Optom. Physiol. Opt.*, **57**, 808–14.

Cullen, A.P. and Chou, B.R. (1984). Blue free fundus examination. *Can. J. Optom.*, **46**, 153–6.

Cullen, A.P., Chou, B.R., Hall, M.G., and Jang, S.E. (1984). Ultraviolet B damages corneal endothelium. *Am. J. Optom. Physiol. Optics.*, **61**, 473–8.

Curtin, T.L. and Boyden, D.G. (1968). Reflected laser beam causing accidental burn of the retina. *Am. J. Ophthalmol.*, **65**, 188–9.

Daily, L., Wakim, K.G., Herrick, J.F. *et al.* (1952). The effects of microwave diathermy on the eye of the rabbit. *Am. J. Ophthalmol.*, **35**, 1001–17.

Deutsch, T.A. and Feller, D.B. (1985). *Paton and Goldberg's management of ocular injuries*, (2nd edn). W.B. Saunders Co., London.

Duke-Elder, S. (ed.) (1972). *System of ophthalmology—injuries*, Vol. XIV, Parts 1 and 2. Henry Kimpton, London.

Edbrooke, C.M. and Edwards, C. (1967). Industrial radiation cataract: the hazards and the protective measures. *Ann. Occup. Hyg.*, **10**, 293.

English, W.P. (1973). Eye protection for welders. *J. Am. Soc. Saf. Eng.*, **July**, 39–43.

Fox, S.L. (1973). *Industrial and occupational ophthalmology*. C.C. Thomas, Illinois.

Goldman, H. (1935). The genesis of the cataract of the glass blower. *Am. J. Ophthalmol.*, **18**, 590.

Good, G.W. and Schoessler, J.P. (1988). Chronic solar radiation exposure and endothelial polymegethism. *Curr., Eye Res.*, **7**, 157–62.

Grant, W.M. (ed.) (1974). *Toxicology of the eye*, (2nd edn). C.C. Thomas, Illinois.

Ham, W.T. Jr., Clarke, A.M., Geeraets, W.J., Cleary, S.F., Mueller, H.A., and Williams, R.C. (1970). The eye problems in laser safety. *Arch. Environ. Health*, **20**, 156–60.

Ham, W.T., Mueller, H.A., Ruffolo, J.J., Guerry, D., and Guerry, R.K. (1982). Action spectrum for retinal injury from near ultraviolet radiation in the aphakic monkey. *Am. J. Ophthalmol.*, **93**, 299–306.

Harding, J.J. and Dilley, K.J. (1976). Structural protein of the mammalian lens: a review with emphasis on changes in development, aging and cataract. *Exp. Eye Res.*, **22**, 1–73.

Harwerth, R.S. and Sperling, H.G. (1971). Prolonged colour blindness induced by intense spectral lights in Rhesus monkeys. *Science* (New York), **174**, 520–3.

Hayes, B.P. and Fisher, R.F. (1979). Influence of prolonged period of low dosage X-rays on the optic and ultrastructural appearance of cataract of the human lens. *Br. J. Ophthalmol.*, **63**, 457–64.

Henkes, H.E. and Zuidema, H. (1975). Accidental laser coagulation of the central fovea. *Ophthalmologica*, **171**, 15–25.

Heriot, W.J. (1985). Light and the retinal pigment epithelium: the link in senile macular degeneration? In *Hazards of light, myths and realities*, (ed. J. Cronly-Dillan, E.S. Rosen, and J. Marshall), pp. 187–96. Pergamon Press, Oxford.

Hiller, R., Giacometti, L., and Yuen, K. (1977). Sunlight and cataract: an epidemiological investigation. *Am. J. Epidemiol.*, **105**, 450–9.

Hollows, F. and Moran, D. (1981). Cataract—the ultra-violet risk factor. *Lancet*, **2**, 1249–50.

Hughes, W.F. Jr. (1946). Alkali burns of the eye II. Clinical and pathological course. *Arch. Ophthalmol.*, **36**, 189–214.

Hunter, D. (1975). *The diseases of occupations*, (5th edn). Hodder and Stoughton, London.

Jacobson, J.H. and McLean, J.M. (1965). Accidental laser retinal burns. *Arch. Ophthalmol.*, **74**, 882.

James, R.H., Bostrom, R.G., Remark, D., and Sliney, D.H. (1988). Handheld ophthalmoscopes for hazards analysis: an evaluation. *Appl. Opt.*, **27**, 5072–6.

Karai, I. and Horiguchi, S. (1984). Pteryguim in welders. *Br. J. Ophthalmol.*, **68**, 347–9.

Klintworth, G.K. (1972). Chronic actinic keratopathy—a condition associated with conjunctival elastosis (pingeculae) and typified by characteristic extracellular concretions. *Am. J. Pathol.*, **67**, 327–48.

Kossol, J., Cole, C., and Dayhaw-Barker, P. (1983). Spectral irradiances of and maximal permissible exposures to two indirect ophthalmoscopes. *Am. J. Optom. Physiol. Optics.*, **60**, 616–21.

Kraff, M.C., Saunders, D.R., Jampol, L.M., and Lieberman, H.L. (1985). Effect of ultraviolet filtering intraocular lens on cystoid macular edema. *Ophthalmol.*, **92**, 366–9.

Kuwabara, T. and Gorn, R.A. (1968). Retinal damage by visible light: an electron microscopic study. *Arch. Ophthalmol.*, **79**, 69–78.

Langely, R.K., Mortimer, C.B., and McCullough, C. (1960). The experimental production of cataracts by exposure to heat and light. *Arch. Ophthalmol.*, **63**, 473.

Lanum, J. (1978). The damaging effect of the light on the retina. Empirical findings, theoretical and practical implications. *Surv. Ophthalmol.*, **22**, 221–49.

Lerman, S. (1980*a*). *Radiant energy and the eye.* Macmillan Publishing Co. Inc., New York.

Lerman, S. (1980*b*). Human ultraviolet radiation cataracts. *Ophthalmic Res.*, **12**, 303–14.

Lerman, S. (1983). An experimental and clinical evaluation of lens transparency and aging. *J. Gerontol.*, **38**, 293–301.

Lerman, S. (1985). Ocular photoxicity. In *Recent advances in ophthalmology*, (ed. S.I. Davidson and F.T. Fraunfelder). Churchill Livingstone, London.

Lerman, S. (1987). Light induced changes in ocular tissues. In *Clinical light damage to the eye*, (ed. D. Miller). Springer Verlag, New York.

Lerman, S., Megaw, J., and Willis, I. (1980). Potential ocular complications of PUVA therapy and their prevention. *J. Invest. Dermatol.*, **74**, 197–9.

Lipman, R.M., Tripathi, B.J., and Tripathi, R.C. (1988). Cataract induced by microwave and ionizing radiation. *Surv. Ophthalmol.*, **33**, 200–10.

Mackenzie, F., Hirst, L., Battistutta, D., and Green, A. (1992). Risk analysis in the development of pterygia. *Ophthalmal.*, **99**, 644–50.

Mainster, M.A. (1987). Light and macular degeneration: a biophysical and clinical perspective. *Eye*, **1**, 304–10.

Mainster, M.A., White T.J., and Allen, R.G. (1970). Spectral dependance of retinal damage produced by intense light sources. *J. Optom. Soc. Am.*, **60**, 848–55.

Mainster, M.A., Timberlake, G.T., Webb, R.H., and Hughes, G.W. (1982). Scanning laser ophthalmoscopy. *Ophthalmology*, **89**, 852–7.

Mainster, M.A., Ham, W.T. Jr., and Delori, F.C. (1983*a*). Potential retinal hazards—instrument and environmental light sources. *Ophthalmology*, **90**, 927–32.

Mainster, M.A., Sliney, D.H., Belcher III, C.D., and Buzney, S.M. (1983*b*). Laser photodisruptors. Damage mechanisms, instrument design safety. *Ophthalmology*, **90**, 927–32.

Marshall, J. (1985). Radiation and the ageing eye. *Ophthal. Physiol. Opt.*, **5**, 241–63.

Marshall, J., Mellerio, J., and Palmer, D.A. (1972). Damage to pigeon retinae by moderate illumination from fluorescent lamps. *Exp. Eye Res.*, **14**, 164–9.

Marshall, J., Trokel, S., Rothery, S., and Krueger R.R. (1986). A comparative study of corneal incisions induced by diamond and steel knives and two ultra-violet radiations from an excimer laser. *Br. J. Ophthalmol.*, **70**, 482–501.

Merriam, G.R. Jr. and Focht, E.F. (1957). A clinical study of radiational cataracts and the relationship to dose. *Am. J. Roentgenol.*, **77**, 759–85.

Merriam, G.R. Jr. and Focht, E.F. (1962). A clinical and experimental study of the effect of single and divided doses of radiation on cataract production. *Trans. Am. Ophthalmol. Soc.*, **60**, 35–52.

Merriam, G.R. Jr., Szechter, A., and Focht, E.F. (1972). The effects of ionizing radiation on the eye. *Radiat. Ther. Oncal.*, **6**, 346–62.

Millodot, M. and Earlam, R.A. (1984). Sensitivity of the cornea after exposure to ultra-violet light. *Ophthalmic Res.*, **16**, 325–8.

Minassian, D.C., Mehra, V., and Jones, B.R. (1984). Dehydrational crises from severe diarrhoea or heat stroke and risk of cataract. *Lancet*, **1**, 751–3.

Minatoya, H.K. (1978). Eye injuries from exploding car batteries. *Arch. Ophthalmol.*, **96**, 477–81.

Moon, M.E.L. and Robertson, I.F. (1983). Retrospective study of alkali burns of the eye. *Aust. J. Ophthalmol.*, **11**, 281–6.

Moran, D.J. and Hollows, F.C. (1984). Pterygium and ultraviolet light: a positive correlation. *Br. J. Ophthalmol.*, **68**, 343–6.

Morgan, S.J. (1987) Chemical burns of the eye— causes and management. *Br. J. Ophthalmol.*, **71**, 854–7.

Noell, W.K., Walker, V.S., Kang, B.S., and Bergman, S. (1966). Retinal damage by light in rats. *Invest. Ophthalmol. Vis. Sci.*, **5**, 450–73.

Norm, M.S. (1982). Spheroid degeneration, pingecula, and pterygium among Arabs in the Red Sea Territory, Jordan. *Acta Ophthalmol.* (kbh), **60**, 949–54.

Novak, J.F. (1970). Ocular trauma in industry. *J. Occup. Med.*, **12**, 287–90.

Novitskaya, V.V. and Novitski, I.Y. (1983). Two cases of ocular damage from lightning. *Vestn. Ofialmol.*, **100**, 71–2.

O'Connor Davies, P.H. (1981). *The actions and uses of ophthalmic drugs* (2nd edn). Butterworth-Heinemann Ltd, London.

O'Steen, W.K., Shear, C.R., and Anderson, K.V. (1972). Retinal damage after exposure to visible light: a light and electron microscopic study. *Am. J. Anat.*, **134**, 5–21.

Palva, M. and Palkama, A. (1978). Ultrastructural lens damage in X-ray induced cataract of the rat. *Acta Ophthalmol.*, **56**, 587–98.

Paterson, C.A. and Pfister, R.R. (1974). Intraocular pressure changes after alkali burns. *Arch. Ophthalmol.*, **91**, 211–18.

Penner, R. and McNair, J.N. (1966). Eclipse blindness: a report of an epidemic in the military population in Hawaii. *Am. J. Ophthalmol.*, **61**, 1452–7.

Pfister, R.R. (1983). Chemical injuries to the eye. *Ophthalmology*, **90**, 1246– 53.

Pfister, R.R., Haddox, J.L., and Patterson, C.A. (1982). The efficacy of sodium citrate in the treatment of severe alkali burns of the eye is influenced by the route of administration. *Cornea*, **1**, 205–11.

Pitts, D.G. (1978). The ocular effects of ultraviolet light. *Am. J. Optom. Physiol. Optics.*, **55**, 19–35.

Pitts, D.G. (1981). Threat of ultraviolet radiation to the eye—how to protect against it. *J. Am. Optom. Assoc.*, **52**, 949–57.

Pitts, D. and Tredici, T. (1971). The effects of ultra-violet light radiation on the eye. *Am. Ind. Hyg. Assoc. J.*, **32**, 231–46.

Pitts, D.G. and Cullen, A.P. (1981). Determination of infra red radiation levels for acute ocular cataractogenesis. *Graefes Arch. Klin. Exp. Ophthalmol.*, **217**, 285.

Plesch, A., Klingbeil, U., and Bille, J. (1987). Digital laser scanning fundus camera. *Appl. Optics*, **26**, 1480–6.

Porter, W.J. (1961). Emergency treatment. *Ophthalmic Opt.*, **1**, 483–5 *et seq.*

Porter, W.J. (1966). Drugs in everyday practice. *Ophthalmic. Opt.*, **6**, 491–8, 507.

Rathkey, A.S. (1965). Accidental laser burn of the macula. *Arch. Ophthalmol.*, **74**, 346–8.

Richardson, A.W., Duane, T.D., and Hies, H.M. (1951). Experimental cataract produced by 3 centimetre pulsed microwave irradiations. *Arch. Ophthalmol.*, **45**, 382–6.

Rodger, F.C. (1973). Clinical findings, course and progress of Bietti's corneal degeneration in the Dahlak Islands. *Br. J. Ophthalmol.*, **57**, 657–64.

Sachsenweger, R. (1980). *Illustrated handbook of ophthalmology*. Wright and Sons Ltd, Bristol.

Schwan, H.P. and Piersol, G.M. (1954). The absorption of electromagnetic energy in body tissues. *Am. J. Phys. Med.*, **33**, 371–404.

Sliney, D.H. and Wolbarsht, M.L. (1980). Safety standards and measurement techniques for high intensity light sources. *Vis. Res.*, **20**, 1133–41.

Stewart-DeHaan, P.J., Creighton, M.O., Larsen, L.E. *et al.* (1985). In vitro studies of microwave-induced cataract: Reciprocity between exposure duration and dose rate for pulsed microwaves. *Exp. Eye. Res.*, **40**, 1–13.

Sykes, S.M., Robinson, W.G., Waxler, M., and Kuwabara, T. (1981). Damage to the monkey retina by broad spectrum fluorescent light. *Invest. Ophthalmol. Vis. Sci.*, **20**, 425–34.

Tier, H. (1984). Toxicological effects on the eyes at work. *Acta Ophthalmol.*, **Suppl. 161**, 60–5.

Trokel, S.L., Srinivasan, R., and Braren, B. (1983). Excimer laser surgery of the cornea. *Am. J. Ophthalmol.*, **96**, 710–15.

Tso, M.O. and La Piana, F.G. (1975). The human fovea after sun gazing. *Trans. Am. Acad. Ophthalmol. Otolaryngol.*, **79**, 788–95.

Van Johnson, E., Kline, L.B., and Skalka, H.W. (1987). Electrical cataracts: a case report and review of the literature. *Ophthalmic Surg.*, **18**, 283–5.

Van Ummerson, C.A. and Cogan, F.C. (1965). Experimental microwave cataracts: age as a factor in induction of cataracts in the rabbit. *Arch. Envir. Health*, **11**, 177–8.

Weale, R.A. (1983). Senile cataract: the case against light. *Ophthalmology*, **90**, 420–3.

Webb, R.H., Hughes, G.W., and Delori, F.C. (1987). Confocal scanning laser ophthalmoscope. *Appl. Optics*, **26**, 1492–9.

Williams, D.B., Monahan, J.P., Nicholson, W.J., and Aldrich, J.J. (1955). Biological effects and studies on microwave radiation; time and power thresholds for production of lens opacities by 12.3 cm microwaver. *Arch. Ophthalmol.*, **54**, 863–74.

Wittenberg, S. (1986). Solar radiation and the eye: a review of knowledge relevant to eyecare. *Am. J. Optom. Physiol. Optics*, **63**, 676–89.

Woo, T.Y. (1985). Lenticular psoralen photoproducts in cataracts of PUVA-treated psoriatic patients. *Acta Dermatol.*, **121**, 1307–8.

Young, R.W. (1988). Solar radiation and age related macular degeneration. *Surv. Ophthalmol.*, **32**, 252–69.

Zigman, S. (1983). The role of sunlight in human cataract formation. *Surv. Ophthalmol.*, **27**, 317–25.

Zigman, S. and Vaughn, R. (1974). Effects of near UV light on the lens and retinas of mice. *Invest. Ophthalmol. Vis. Sci.*, **13**, 462–5.

Zweng, H.C. (1967). Accidental Q-switched laser lesion of the human macula. *Arch. Ophthalmol.*, **78**, 596–9.

Further reading

Deutsch, T.A. and Feller, B. (1985). *Paton and Goldberg's management of ocular injuries*. W.B. Saunders, Philadelphia.

Miller, D. (ed.) (1987). *Clinical light damage to the eye*. Springer-Verlag, New York.

Roper-Hall, M.J. (1987). *Eye emergencies*. Churchill Livingstone, Edinburgh.

Sliney, D. and Wolbarsht, M. (1980). *Safety with lasers and other optical sources. A comprehensive handbook*. Plenum Press, London.

Waxler, M. and Hitchings, V.M. (1986). *Optical radiation and visual health*. CRC Press Inc., Florida.

6. Construction of eye-protectors[*]

Potential ocular hazards, such as flying particles and chemical splashes, should be eliminated or controlled at source. However, if this is not possible, the appropriate type of eye-protection must be provided and worn. Screens or fixed shields can be used alone or in addition to eye-protectors to guard against potential hazards. People are now becoming more aware of the need to protect their eyes and eye-protectors should not only be provided to fulfil legal obligations at work but also for the many other leisure activities, such as DIY, ski-ing, squash, and ice hockey.

Ideally, an eye-protector must be:

(1) constructed to provide the necessary protection against the hazard for which it is designed, e.g. flying particles or radiation;

(2) comfortable during wear and not liable to steam up;

(3) light-weight and not interfere with movements;

(4) easily cleaned;

(5) readily replaced at reasonable cost;

(6) constructed so that it does not impair visual function;

(7) durable, non-flammable, and non-irritant to the skin;

(8) of suitable optical quality;

(9) cosmetically acceptable;

(10) compatible with other protective devices, such as ear and respiratory protective equipment.

Eye-protectors may be in the form of spectacles, goggles (cup or box), screens, or visors supported by a headband, or in the form of a helmet. Figure 6.1 shows some of the types of eye-protectors available.

The lenses for these eye-protectors may be made of the following materials:

* This chapter is a revised version of North, R.V. and Earlam, R.A. (1988). Eye-protection. In *Optometry* (ed. K. Edwards and R. Llewellyn), pp. 523–34. Butterworth-Heinemann, Oxford.

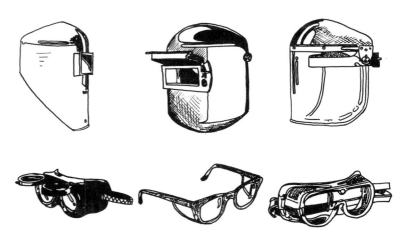

Fig. 6.1 Different types of eye-protectors.

(1) glass—heat and special heat-toughened, chemically-toughened, and laminated;
(2) plastics—polymethylmethacrylate (PMMA), allyl diglycol carbonate (CR39), polycarbonate, and cellulose acetate;
(3) wire gauze.

Frames or lens housing may be made of:

(1) metal—nickel;
(2) plastics—cellulose acetate, cellulose acetate butyrate (CAB), polyamide (e.g. nylon), and polycarbonate.

Lens materials

Heat-toughened glass

Glass is a fragile and brittle material, which breaks into very sharp splinters. It is, therefore, unsuitable for an impact-resistant eye-protector, unless it is heat- or chemically toughened.

Heat-toughened glass lenses are usually made from spectacle crown glass. The toughening process begins when the edged-lens is placed into a furnace and heated to 637 °C for 50–300 s (Collins 1983). The time spent in the oven depends on the weight, size, and average thickness of the lens. After heating, the lens is withdrawn and cooled rapidly, usually by a jet of cold air. The sudden cooling creates a state of compression at the lens surface and a state of tension in the lens mass. This produces a compression-tension coat, often referred to as the compression envelope. As glass is stronger in compression than tension, the compression envelope improves the impact resistance. After the lenses have been manufactured they are fitted into the frame/housing.

Advantages
1. Heat toughening is a compratively quick process.
2. It does not need skilled labour.

3. The equipment needed is inexpensive and requires little bench space.

4. It is a relatively cheap process.

Disadvantages

1. Prescription lenses over + 5.00 D are not ideal for toughening, as the bulk of glass requires prolonged heating. This can cause warping, which degrades the optical qualities. Warping can be seen easily when viewing the focimeter image produced through the reading portion of fused bifocals. Lenses of over − 5.00 D have poor impact resistance due to the relatively small centre substance (Collins 1983).

2. A heat-toughened lens will always be thicker than an untoughened lens of equivalent power. However, in the UK, the Pilkington thin lens technique has produced good performance safety prescription lenses with a minimum centre thickness of only 1.9 mm and 1.4 mm minumum edge thickness (Tunnacliffe 1989). Compare this with 2.4 mm centre substance and 1.8 mm edge thickness of conventionally heat-toughened lenses; these thin lenses are lighter. The Norville Optical Company Ltd supply these thinner toughened glass lenses in a power range from +/− 8.00 D; they meet the basic grade of BS 2092 (1987).

3. Impact resistance is markedly reduced by scratches and other surface abrasions and lenses that conformed to BS 2092 when first received from the factory will not retain the same level of impact resistance throughout life. As the lens surface will naturally become scratched with use, lenses should be inspected regularly, and replaced when distinct scratches are present (Silberstein 1964).

4. The heat-toughening process has an adverse effect on the photochromic salts present in photochromic lenses. It reduces the range of activity and the lens does not lighten to the original transmission. To restore most of this activity it is necessary to apply a secondary annealing process.

5. When heat-toughened glass lenses are viewed through a polariscope or strain tester, a shadow or strain pattern can be seen; the Maltese cross-shape is typical. This pattern is induced during the heat-toughening process when the lens is cooled. The method of thin lens toughening does not give the characteristic Maltese cross stress pattern, but shows a shadow pattern that varies from lens to lens.

Chemically toughened glass

This is a more recent method of toughening glass, which is very popular in Europe. As with heat toughening the impact resistance is formed by the creation of a compression-tension coat. In this case, however, it is produced by a chemical process. The lenses are first preheated and then lowered into a potassium nitrate solution at 470 °C for 16 h (Jalie 1984). The compression coat is produced by exchanging the larger potassium ions present in the solution for the smaller sodium ions present in the glass. As this treatment occurs on the surface of the glass only, it produces a very thin, but very tough, compression coat (100 µm thick). For photochromic lens toughening the solution normally used is 40 per cent potassium nitrate and 60 per cent sodium nitrate at a reduced temperature of 400 °C. This process does not generally affect the photochromic activity of lenses.

Advantages

1. Although chemically toughened lenses are thinner than heat-toughened lenses, they have been shown to possess a greater impact resistance.
2. Chemically toughened glass has a greater impact resistance to large particles/missiles than conventionally heat-toughened glass (Woodward and Melling 1977).
3. Chemical toughening is suitable for many lenses of stock thickness; specially surfaced lenses are therefore required only infrequently.
4. The toughening process takes the same time for all types of lenses.
5. The temperature required for chemical toughening is lower than that used in the heat treatment of lenses. Warping is therefore not a problem.

Disadvantages

1. Chemical toughening is an expensive process, as it requires equipment that must withstand the chemicals and the temperatures involved.
2. It is not ideally suited for crown glass—a special type of glass is needed for the best results. This glass is more expensive.
3. Scratches on the lens surface reduce the impact resistance because of damage to the very thin compression coat (Woodward and Melling 1977).
4. It is difficult to determine whether the lens has been toughened, as there is neither a stress pattern nor a conventional method that will provide this information.

When chemically or heat-toughened glass lenses fracture they usually show a radial fracture pattern, although concentric cracks can also occur (Fig. 6.2). Therefore, only a few splinters of glass are produced and the fragments tend to stay in the spectacle frame.

Laminated glass

Laminated glass lenses are made by the adhesion of two layers of crown glass to an inner layer of plastics material. This type of lens has an impact resistance only slightly higher than crown glass. If it shatters, the glass is supposed to stick to the plastics inter-layer. However, large, low velocity missiles may result in slivers of glass from the back glass surface injuring the eye.

Plastics

Plastics lenses have many advantages over glass and are widely used as eye-protectors, especially where impact resistance is required. The advantages of plastics lenses are (Jalie 1984):

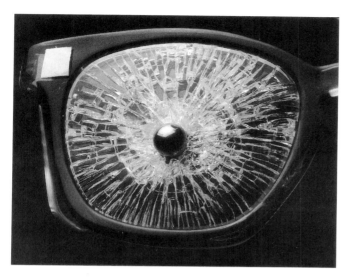

Fig. 6.2 Fracture pattern of a heat-toughened lens. The lens was impacted with a steel ball bearing, which did not penetrate it (© B. Tarr).

1. They offer greater impact resistance, particularly against high velocity particles.
2. Scratches on the lens surface do not obviously affect the impact resistance.
3. If the lens is fractured, the fragments tend to be larger and relatively blunt.
4. The weight is about 50 per cent of that of a glass lens of equivalent power (Fig. 6.3).
5. A plastics lens can be thinner than a glass lens of equivalent power, as it may not be necessary to thicken the lens as much to maintain the impact resistance.
6. Plastics generally withstand molten metal splashes and hot sparks better than glass, as the metal does not fuse with the lens surface.
7. Plastic lenses are less susceptible to condensation, which is due to the lower thermal conductivity.
8. Plastics offer greater protection against UV radiation.

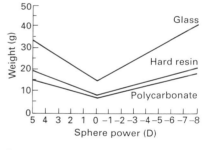

Fig. 6.3 The weight of different lens materials (after Herbert 1984, courtesy of Gentex Corporation Ltd and *Optical World*).

Disadvantages

1. The lens surface is easily abraded because the material is soft; it needs an abrasion-resistant coating. Unfortunately, this has been shown to reduce the impact resistance of some lenses.
2. The refractive indices for plastics lenses range from 1.49 to 1.60. The higher index is usually accompanied by a lower V-value (Abbe number). The V-value is the reciprocal of the dispersive power for the material. In general, the greater the V-value the better the material optically, as the chromatic aberrations produced decreases as V increases (Jalie 1984).

Polymethyl methacrylate (PMMA) and Columbia Resin 39 (CR39)

PMMA (ICI perspex) was the first plastics material used in the UK for prescription lenses (Igard/Igard Z). These lenses have, to a large extent, been replaced by the thermosetting plastics CR39 (allyl diglycol carbonate). CR39 offers a greater impact resistance than PMMA but, when the lens breaks, it produces sharper fragments. However, both of these materials are suitable for eye-protectors. Lenses can be made up as a combination of PMMA and CR39. Prescription lenses for eye-protectors are commonly made from CR39, which can easily be tinted if required, using a dying technique. This method of tinting cannot be applied to PMMA lenses, as it causes deformation of the lens.

Polycarbonate

This has the highest impact resistance of all lens materials. Unfortunately, it has a very soft surface, which is easily abraded. To avoid abrasion a quartz coating is often used. Polycarbonate is commonly used for plano eye-protectors—where lenses and front are made in one piece by injection moulding. Its popularity for use as a prescription lens material in eye-protectors is increasing, particularly as it is now accepted for BS 2092.2 (1987).

Advantages

1. Polycarbonate has a much greater impact resistance than heat-toughened glass. If the lens does fracture upon impact it cracks; it does not break into particles.
2. Silica-coated lenses are more abrasion-resistant than uncoated lenses.
3. There is no age-related warping, chipping, or discoloration.
4. Polycarbonate is the lightest lens material available (specific gravity 1.2).
5. Polycarbonate has a fairly high refractive index (1.586).
6. The material absorbs UV radiation.

Disadvantages

1. Compared with glass or CR39, the surface quality of polycarbonate is poor.
2. Polycarbonate lenses can be tinted only by a vacuum coating process.
3. The V-value is poor (30) and causes colour fringes. This is most marked when viewing through the periphery of the lens, especially with high power prescriptions.
4. Abrasion-resistant coatings can decrease the impact resistance from 244 m/s to 152 m/s (Greenberg et al. 1985).

Cellulose acetate

This has a relatively poor impact resistance, compared with polycarbonate and therefore is used only for basic eye-protectors. However, it does have good resistance to chemicals and is more often used for chemical visors and box goggles.

Wire gauze

Goggles made from wire gauze have a very good impact resistance but are generally not accepted, because they degrade the visual function and give no protection against splashes of molten metal, etc.

Testing procedures of protective lenses

The lenses used in eye-protectors must be tested to establish whether they are suitable for the specific hazard for which they were designed. The following factors may be assessed:

(1) impact resistance;

(2) surface hardness;

(3) chemical resistance;

(4) thermostability;

(5) flammability;

(6) resistance to hot particles;

(7) radiosensitivity.

Impact resistance

The impact resistance of a lens can be influenced by:

(1) abrasions/scratches on the lens surface;

(2) size and speed of missile/particle;

(3) lens thickness;

(4) type of material.

The impact resistance of all types of lenses may be reduced when the surface has been abraded. There are two modes of failure, which partly depend upon the size of the missile. Large particles (> 16 mm) hitting a lens, cause it to bend and so the failure is initiated on the back surface. Therefore, any scratches that occur on the front surface due to wear and tear will not have a significant effect on the impact resistance. Smaller particles do not cause the lens to bend upon impact, so the fracture is generally initiated on the front surface. In this case the impact resistance to smaller particles will be reduced for all types of lenses when the front surface has been abraded (Welsh et al. 1974). The impact resistance was reduced by 20 per cent for heat-toughened lenses, and by more than 30 per cent for chemically toughened lenses (Woodward and Melling 1977).

In general, as the missile size decreases, the lens' impact resistance (measured as the fracture velocity) increases (Wigglesworth 1971a). Table 6.1 shows the mean fracture velocities of lens materials for different sizes of missiles. When a 3 mm heat-toughened glass lens is hit by a large missile (19.1–28.6 mm) it demonstrates more impact resistance than a CR39 lens of similar thickness. However, when the missile is small (3.2–6.3 mm) the CR39 lens performs best. It has also been shown that for small missiles (< 6.4 mm) chemically toughened lenses are not as

Table 6.1 Mean fracture velocities of lens materials (m/s) (after Wigglesworth, E.C. (1972). A comparative assessment of eye-protective devices and proposed system of acceptance testing and grading. *Am. J. Optom. A.A.A.O.*, **49**, 287–304. Copyright The Am. Acad. of Optom; and Greenberg *et al*. 1985)

Lens material	Thickness of lens (mm)	Missile diameter (mm)		
		25.4	6.5	3.2
CR39	3	6.6	49	88
CR39	2	5.0	39	63
Polymethyl methacrylate	3	4.5	34	58
Toughened glass	3	7.6	18	29
Toughened glass	2	3.7	12	23
Untoughened glass	3	3.1	12	23
Laminated glass	3	2.2	12	25
Polycarbonate				
coated*	3		152	
uncoated*	3		244	

Data from Wigglesworth (1972) and * Greenberg *et al*. 1985.

resistant as heat-toughened lenses, whilst for larger missiles (> 6.4 mm) they have a slightly superior performance (Woodward and Melling 1977).

As the lens thickness increases, the impact resistance also increases; impact resistance also increases slightly as the lens is curved. The strength increases with increasing base curve (6.00–10.00 D) with both heat-toughened and CR39 lenses (Wiggleworth 1971*b*).

The type of material used for an eye-protector gives an indication of the mean fracture velocity that can be tolerated. Figure 6.4 shows the

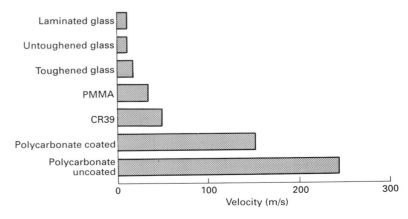

Fig. 6.4 Fracture velocity of a 3 mm thick sample of different lens materials when struck by a 6.5 mm diameter steel ball (data from Table 6.1).

fracture velocity for some of the materials available. The samples were all of the same thickness and were struck by a 6.5 mm steel ball. Polycarbonate offers the greatest fracture resistance of all lens materials (Welsh *et al.* 1974; Greenberg *et al.* 1985).

Hardness

There have been many efforts to study the problems associated with surface abrasion, not all of which fully represent the natural wear and tear. There are distinct advantages in coating plastics lenses, particularly polycarbonate, which is a soft thermoplastic. A thinly coated (5 μm) polycarbonate lens is superior to an uncoated CR39 lens.

Chemical resistance

Glass lenses are resistant to most chemicals. Plastics, however, may show crazing and surface clouding with some strong chemical solutions. CR39 has quite good chemical resistance and is frequently used for chemical visors and box goggle windows.

Thermostability

Polycarbonate and polymethyl methacrylate are prone to distort more readily than glass. PMMA softens at 80 °C, CR39 at 100 °C and polycarbonate at 120 °C (Jalie 1984).

Flammability

All the plastic materials are flammable. However, as their ignition temperatures are high, they are considered safe for use.

Resistance to hot particles

Eye-protectors must be able to withstand hot particles impinging upon them, as can occur in such processes as grinding or welding. A glass surface is very easily pitted by these particles, as they fuse with the surface. Plastics, on the other hand, do not pit easily (Fig. 6.5). This is possibly due to the elasticity of the surface when heated by the particle.

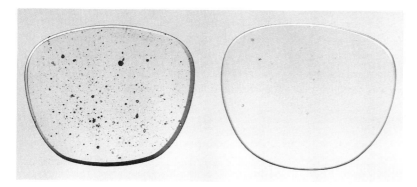

Fig. 6.5 Resistance to hot particles by a glass lens (left) and a CR39 plastic lens (right). After equal exposure to spatter from an arc welder the glass lens is considerably more pitted than the CR39 plastic lens (© B. Tarr).

Radiosensitivity

This should be considered in cases where a lens has broken and particles have penetrated the eye. In this situation a series of X-rays taken from different angles may locate the particle/s. Material that is nearly invisible to X-rays the particle will be most difficult to locate; glass fragments can be observed by X-ray techniques when they are not too small (> 0.5 mm) but plastics particles are very difficult to find (Collins 1983).

A summary of the properties of the various materials used for lenses in eye-protectors is given in Table 6.2.

Materials for lens housing

The lens housing may be made of metal (e.g. a nickel alloy) or plastics (e.g. polycarbonate, polyamide, and cellulose acetate/butyrate). These materials may be used in the manufacture of:

(1) spectacle frames;
(2) goggles—both cup and box type;
(3) face shields;
(4) helmets.

Spectacle frames

Protective spectacle frames may be manufactured by three methods (Fatt 1977):

1. Front cut from a flat sheet of plastics material. Frames manufactured by this process are generally used for prescription eye-protectors and are made from cellulose acetate.
2. Frame formed by injection moulding from plastics granules. This technique again uses cellulose acetate for frames, which are generally glazed with prescription lenses. Polyamide (e.g. nylon) or polycarbonate is often used for plano eye-protectors.
3. Frames made from wire (e.g. nickel type). These frames have been shown to cause more damage upon impact than a plastics frame. Injury may occur when a blow forces the frame against the upper brow and cheek. Frames with the adjustable toggle pads can cause more injury to the nose than those with a plastics bridge.

Particular concern has been expressed about the use of metal frames for prescription eye-protectors for the following reasons:

1. The screws quickly work loose, notably the rim securing screws.
2. Accurate glazing of the lens is critical. If the lens is too small it may fall out; if too large it may induce stresses at the edge of the lens.
3. Metal frames have narrower rims than plastics frames, which makes the glazing of high power lenses more difficult.

Recommendations relating to the use of metal frames (Grundy 1982) are as follows:

Table 6.2 A comparison of the major properties of glazing materials for eye-protectors (modified from Grundy 1987, courtesy of J. Grundy and *Optometry Today*)

Material	Impact resistance		Hardness	Chemical resistance	Thermostability	Fracture pattern	Resistance to hot particles	Weight
	Large missile	Small missile						
Glass								
Heat-toughened	Good	Good	Good	Very good	Very good	Fair	Poor	Heaviest
Chemically toughened	Good	Poor	Good	Very good	Very good	Fair	Poor	Heavy
Laminated	Fair	Fair	Good	Good	Fair	Poor	Poor	Heavy
Plastics								
PMMA	Fair	Fair	Poor	Good	Fair	Good	Very good	Light
CR39	Good	Good	Fair	Good	Good	Fair	Good	Light
Cellulose acetate	Good	Good	Poor	Good	Fair	Good	Fair	Light
Polycarbonate (coated)	Very good	Very good	Poor	Fair	Good	Very good	Good	Light

1. Rim screws should be secured by a lock nut, peening, or adhesives that bond the thread.
2. Plastics lenses should be used instead of glass.
3. Separate rim-securing screws and side hinge screws should be used.

Side shields for spectacle frames

These must not restrict the wearer's field of vision. They should therefore be made of a transparent material, which does not discolour with age. Injection-moulded side shields are best, as their shape does not alter (unlike those made from a flat sheet, which tend to warp). Any warping of the side shield will produce gaps between the shield and the front, allowing particles direct access to the eye. Ideally, side shields should be made of injection-moulded polycarbonate material. They may also be made from wire gauze or perforated plastics, to allow a better air flow and so to prevent condensation.

The main advantage of spectacle eye-protectors is that they can be made to fit well, as there is a range of sizes available. Spectacles are not suitable for BS 2092 (1987) grade 1 impact protection, dusts, molten metal or liquid droplets, or splashes.

Afocal one piece eye-protector

These are usually moulded in one piece from polycarbonate. This type of protector has the advantage that the lenses cannot be dislodged, as may occur with a spectacle frame. They are suitable for emmetropes, but are usually manufactured in only one size. As the fit required is different for each person, they do not always fit well. If not fitted correctly, eye-protectors will not provide the necessary protection and eye injury may still occur. Prescription eye-protectors are normally fitted by an optometric practitioner or dispensing optician and should be adjusted carefully on collection. It is most unfortunate that afocal eye-protectors are often handed out by safety officers, who do not have the necessary training or the facilities to fit them.

Afocal eye-protectors are often disliked by employees who do not normally wear spectacles and are therefore worn very reluctantly. The employees' complaints can be listed as follows (Garner 1973):

1. Restricted field of view, due to the frame.
2. Magnification effect. Afocal lenses can give a small magnification, caused by the shape of the lenses (base curve).
3. Reflections from the lens surfaces give rise to unwanted ghost images.
4. Peripheral displacement effects of afocal lenses increase with centre thickness, base curve, and angle of ocular rotation. The vertical displacement effect induced on ocular rotation is only a problem if the lenses of a pair have different base curves.

The uses, advantages, and disadvantages of the two different types of goggles will now be summarized (Rousell 1979; Grunday 1981).

Goggles—cup type

These may be used to provide protection against molten metal, flying particles, dust, etc. A good tight fit to the face is required. The housing is generally made of polyvinyl chloride (PVC).

Advantages

1. They have an adjustable nasal fitting, i.e. distance between rims.
2. Screw rim types allow the lenses to be replaced or exchanged for another type of lens, e.g. tinted or impact resistant.
3. Large bridge aprons are often available to protect the nose.

Disadvantages

1. They cannot normally be worn over prescription spectacles.
2. Ventilation is often poor, which causes the lenses to mist. If present, the ventilation holes must be screened to prevent penetration and blocking by dust or chemicals, etc.
3. They are sometimes uncomfortable, as the cup is hard. The separation of the lenses is often too large, causing an obstruction of central vision.
4. Peripheral vision is restricted.

Goggles—box type

Box type goggles are normally made of PVC, which gives a good fit around the brows and cheeks. The one-piece lens may be of cellulose acetate, polycarbonate, or possibly toughened glass.

Advantages

1. They can normally be worn comfortably over prescription spectacles.
2. They usually have good ventilation.
3. They are light-weight.
4. There is no central obstruction of vision.
5. There is a wide field of view.

Disadvantages

1. The nasal fitting is not adjustable.
2. The one-piece lenses are not always easy to replace and hence the whole eye-protector may have to be discarded.
3. Prescription wearers may sometimes have difficulty in achieving comfort or a proper fit of the goggles over their prescription spectacles.

Face shields

These are usually headband-supported visors that cover the face and neck. They are used to provide protection from flying particles, molten metal, and chemical splashes, and can easily be worn over prescription spectacles or other types of eye-protection, if required. They provide an excellent field of view. The face shield is generally made from either polycarbonate or cellulose acetate. They can also be made so that they can

Table 6.3 Styles of eye-protectors available, BS 7028. (Reproduced with kind permission of B.S.I.) Complete copies can be obtained from BSI Sales, Linford Wood, Milton Keynes, MK14 6LE

British Standard 2092 type of eye-protection	Available style of protection		
	Spectacles/eye shields	Goggles	Face screens
Basic	Yes	Yes	Yes
Grade 2 impact	Yes	Yes	Yes
Grade 1 impact	No	Yes	Yes
Liquid droplets	No	Yes	No
Liquid splashes	No	No	Yes
Dusts	No	Yes	No
Gases	No	Yes	No
Molten metals	No	Yes	Yes
Combination impact/molten metals	No	Yes	Yes
Combination impact/liquid droplets	No	Yes	No
Combination impact/liquid splashes	No	No	Yes
Combination impact dusts	No	Yes	No
Combination impact/gases	No	Yes	No
Welding filters incorporated in equipment to BS 1542	Yes Used for class 1 operations only as given in BS 1542	Yes	Yes also hand-held shields, helmets and fixed shields
Laser eye-protectors	No	Yes	No

be hand-held, e.g. the arc welding screens, which have a filter as the ocular (i.e. a tinted window). Face shields are also used to provide protection in occupations such as motorcycling, cricket, and the security industry.

Helmets

Helmets are commonly worn during welding. They provide protection of the face and neck from intense radiation and spatter. There is an ocular containing a filter to prevent harmful radiation from reaching the eyes. The filter may be designed so that it can be flipped up to expose a clear, impact resistant lens, which can be used for grinding and chipping operations. There are some superior variations of this appliance where the window is fitted with a polarizing cell, which darkens to welding density as soon as the arc is struck. These appliances usually have their own air supply, as the gases from welding rods are toxic.

Table 6.3 shows the different types of eye-protectors and the range of hazards for which they may be used (according to BS 2092 (1987) and BS 1542 (1982)).

Summary

Various types of eye-protectors have been described. These can offer protection against different types of ocular hazards and it is essential that the hazards are correctly identified so that the appropriate eye-protector can be supplied.

References

BS 1542 (1982). *Equipment for eye, face and neck protection against radiation arising during welding and similar operations*. British Standards Institution, London.

BS 2092 (1987). *Eye-protectors for industrial and non-industrial uses*. British Standards Institution, London.

BS 7028 (1988). *Guide to selection, care, maintenance of eye-protectors for industrial and other uses*. British Standards Institution, London.

Collins, M. (1983). *Occupational public health optometry*, pp. 25–41. Queensland Institute of Technology, Brisbane.

Fatt, I. (1977). Is the frame safe? *Mfg. Opt. Int.*, **March**, 109–10.

Garner, L.F. (1973). Optical requirements for personal eye protectors. In *Vision and its protection. A symposium on visual efficiency and eye protection at work*, (ed. E.C. Wigglesworth and B.L. Cole), pp. 77–93. Australian Optometrical Publishing Company, Sydney.

Greenberg, I., Chase, G., and Lamarre, D. (1985). Stastical protocol for impact testing prescription polycarbonate safety lenses. *Optical World*, **March/April**, 7–8.

Grundy, J.W. (1982). Eye protectors constructed with metal spectacle frames. *Ophthal. Optician*, **July 31**, 550–2.

Grundy, J.W. (1987). A diagrammatic approach to occupational optometry and illumination. Part 3. Industrial hazards and eye protection. *Optom. Today*, **Sept 12**, 562–74.

Herbert, S. (1984). The polycarb story could have a happy ending. *Optical World*, **April/May**, 4–8.

Jalie, M. (1984). *The principles of ophthalmic lenses*, (4th edn). Association of Dispensing Opticians, London.

Rousell, D. (1979). *Eye protection*. Publication No. IS126, obtainable from: the Royal Society for the Prevention of Accidents, Cannon House, The Priory, Queensway, Birmingham.

Silberstein, I.W. (1964). The fracture resistance of industrially damaged safety glass lenses. Plano and prescription—an expanded study. *Am. J. Optom. AAAO.*, **41**, 199–220.

Tunnacliffe, A.H. (1989). *Ophthalmic lens data. The complete reference.* J.R. Stallwood & Assoc, West Sussex.

Welsh, K.W., Miller, J.W., Kislin, B., Tredici, T.J., and Rahe, A.J. (1974). Ballistic impact testing of scratched and unscratched ophthalmic lenses. *Am. J. Optom. Physiol. Opt.*, **51**, 304–11.

Wigglesworth, E.C. (1971a). A ballistic assessment of eye protector lens material. *Invest. Ophthal. Vis. Sci.*, **10**, 985–91.

Wigglesworth, E.C. (1971b). The impact resistance of eye protector lens material. *Am. J. Optom. AAAO.*, **48**, 245–61.

Wigglesworth, E.C. (1972). A comparative assessment of eye protective devices and proposed system of acceptance testing and grading. *Am. J. Optom. AAAO.*, **49**, 287–304.

Woodward, A. and Melling, R. (1977). Glass, the basic material. *Ophthal. Optician*, **March 19**, 231–3.

7. Regulations and standards relating to eye-protection

Protection of Eyes Regulations

The Protection of Eyes Regulations were drawn up in 1974 to replace section 49 of the Factories Act (1937). They came into force on 10 April 1975. These regulations give details of listed processes where eyes must be protected, even in situations where people may be at risk although not specifically engaged in the process. Additional legal requirements may be necessary under the terms of the Factories Act (1961), the Protection of Eyes (Amendment) Regulations (1975) (Statutory Instruments 303) and also the Health and Safety at Work etc. Act (1974).

The Protection of Eyes Regulations have increased the number of jobs and processes that require eye-protection, and they also regulate the standards of the eye-protectors. To be able to apply these regulations to any factory where listed processes are carried out, the regulations must be read in conjunction with the Certificates of Approval required by clause 2(2). The Certificates of Approval were made by HM Chief Inspector of Factories and give details of the construction, marking, and particulars that should accompany the various forms of eye-protection (i.e. the relevant British Standards). Certificate No. 1 (HMSO publication F2475) states that eye-protectors, shields, and fixed shields should conform to BS 2092, BS 1542, and BS 679. Certificate No. 2 (HMSO publication F2489) states that protection against lasing sources should conform to BS 4803 (the last standard has recently been superseded by BS 7192).

A brief summary of the clauses of particular importance and their possible implications follow.

Clause 2(2)

This lists and describes the various types of eye-protection:

1. Eye-protectors—goggles, visors, spectacles, or face screen.
2. Shield—helmet or hand shield.
3. Fixed shield—a screen that is either free-standing or fixed to machines, etc.

Table 7.1 Terms used for eye-protectors in the Protection of Eyes Regulations and the corresponding definitions given in the British Standards

Regulations	British Standard
Goggles	Goggles cup type BS 2092, 1542
Visors	Goggles box type BS 2092, 1542
Spectacles	Spectacles BS 2092, 1542
Face screen	Face screen BS 2092
Shields	Face shield BS 1542
	Hand shield BS 1542
	Helmet BS 1542

The terms used in the regulations and the related British Standards are slightly different. Table 7.1 gives the terms used in the regulations and the corresponding definitions given in the appropriate British Standard.

Clauses 5 and 6

These clauses describe the type of protection that should be provided for the various listed processes, e.g. whether eye-protectors can be used or whether shields are required.

There are two schedules:

1. Schedule 1 deals with the protection of persons employed in the specific processes.
2. Schedule 2 deals with the protection of persons at risk from but not actually employed in a specified process.

Clause 7. Eye-protectors—issue and availability

Eye-protectors should be given by the employer into the possession of each person, i.e. they should be issued personally to each employee. The only exception is in the case of persons who are occasionally employed in the specific process, but there should be a sufficient number of well maintained eye-protectors readily available for their use.

Clause 8. Replacement of eye-protectors

When an eye-protector has been provided it must be replaced immediately it is reported as lost, destroyed, defective, or unsuitable for use. This applies to all eye-protectors except prescription spectacles, where the employer must issue a suitable protective device to be worn over the employee's own prescription spectacles, e.g. box type goggle or face screen.

If the employee's type of work changes and they encounter new hazards then the eye-protector must be replaced or supplementary protection must be supplied. The employer must maintain stocks of all the types of eye-protection used so that replacement can be provided immediately when either the employee has reported the need or the employer is aware of the deficiency and need for replacement.

Clause 9. Eye-protectors and shields: construction and marking

Eye-protectors and shields provided in pursuance of these regulations shall:

(a) be suitable for the person for whose use they are provided,

(b) be made in conformity with an approved specification for eye-protectors or shields, as the case may be, being an approved specification for eye-protectors or shields which are appropriate to the specified process in which the said person is employed or from the carrying on of which there is a reasonably foreseeable risk of injury to the eyes of the said person, as the case may be; and

(c) be marked in such a manner and accompanied by such particulars as may be approved in order to indicate the purpose or purposes for which the eye-protectors or shields were designed.

This is an important clause, as it places upon the employer the responsibility for ensuring that the eye-protector and shield is appropriate for the process involved and that they are also suitable for the person employed in that process. The term 'suitable' could be interpreted as meaning an effective and comfortable fit of the eye-protector. Therefore, if afocal or prescription safety spectacles are being provided the bridge size, side length, etc. must be correct to give a proper and comfortable fit. When side shields are present they must be adjusted correctly, or they will not give the required protection.

The phrase 'appropriate to the specified process' has many implications. The nature of the hazard must be assessed correctly, the fitting of the eye protector must be effective and it must be compatible with other protective devices that may also have to be worn, e.g. respirators and ear defenders.

Clause 11. Duties of employed persons

The employees must use the protection that has been provided. They shall take reasonable care of the protective device and not wilfully misuse them/it. They must also report to the employer any loss or damage of, or defect in, the protective device. If a fixed shield is provided an employee shall make full and proper use of it.

Schedule 1

Part 1

This requires approved eye-protectors to be worn by persons employed in any of the 23 specified processes listed below:

1. The blasting or erosion of concrete by means of shot or other abrasive materials.
2. The cleaning of buildings or structures by means of shot or other abrasive materials propelled by compressed air.
3. Cleaning by means of high pressure water jets.

4. The striking of masonry nails by means of a hammer or other hand tool or by means of power-driven portable tool.

5. Any work carried out with a hand held cartridge operated tool, including the operation of loading and unloading live cartridges into a tool, and the handling of such a tool for the purpose of maintenance, repair or examination when the tool is loaded with a live cartridge.

6. The chipping of metal, and the chipping, knocking out, cutting out or cutting off of cold rivets, bolts, nuts, lugs, pins, collars, or similar articles from any structure or plant, or from part of any structure or plant, by means of a hammer, chisel, punch, or similar hand tool, or by means of a power-driven portable tool.

7. The chipping or scurfing of paint, scale, slag, rust, or other corrosion from the surface of metal and other hard materials by means of a hand tool or by means of a power-driven portable tool or by applying articles of metal or such materials to a power driven tool.

8. The use of a high speed metal cutting saw or an abrasive cutting-off wheel or disc, which in either case is power driven.

9. The pouring or skimming of molten metal in foundries.

10. Work at a molten salt bath when the molten surface is exposed.

11. The operation, maintenance, dismantling or demolition of plant or any part of plant, being plant or part of plant which contains, or has contained acids, alkalis, dangerous corrosive substances, whether liquid or solid, or other substances which are similarly injurious to the eyes, and which has not been so prepared (by isolation, reduction of pressure, emptying or otherwise), treated or designed and constructed as to prevent any forseeable risk of injury to the eyes of any person engaged in any such work from any of the said contents.

12. The handling in open vessels or manipulation of acids, alkalis, dangerous corrosive materials, whether liquid or solid, and other substances which are similarly injurious to the eyes, where in any of the foregoing cases there is a reasonably foreseeable risk of injury to the eyes of any person engaged in any such work from drops splashed or particles thrown off.

13. The driving in or on of bolts, pins, collars or similar articles to any structure or plant or to part of any structure or plant by means of a hammer, chisel, punch or similar hand tool or by means of a power-driven portable tool, where in any of the foregoing cases there is a reasonable foreseeable risk of injury to the eyes of any person engaged in the work from particles or fragments thrown off.

14. Injection by high pressure of liquids or solutions into buildings or structures or parts thereof where in the course of any such work there is a reasonably foreseeable risk of injury to the eyes of any person engaged in the work from any such liquids or solutions.

15. The breaking up of metal by means of a hammer, whether power driven or not, or by means of a tup, where in either of the foregoing cases there is reasonably foreseeable risk of injury to the eyes of any person engaged in the work from particles or fragments thrown off.

16. The breaking, cutting, cutting into, dressing, carving or drilling by means of power-driven portable tool or by means of a hammer, chisel, pick or similar hand tool other than a trowel, of any of the following, that is to say—(a) glass, hard plastics, concrete, fired clay, plaster, slag or stone (whether natural or artificial); (b) materials similar to any of the foregoing; (c) articles consisting wholly or partly of any of the foregoing; (d)

stonework, brickwork or blockwork; (e) bricks, tiles or blocks (except blocks made of wood), where in any of the foregoing cases there is a reasonably foreseeable risk of injury to the eyes of any person engaged in the work from particles or fragments thrown off.

17. The use of compressed air to remove swarf, dust, dirt or other particles, where in the course of any such work there is reasonably foreseeable risk of injury to the eyes of any person engaged in the work from particles or fragments thrown off.

18. Work at a furnace containing molten metal, and the pouring or skimming of molten metal in places other than founderies, where there is reasonably foreseeable risk of injury to the eyes of any person engaged in any such work from molten metal.

19. Processes in foundries where there is a reasonably foreseeable risk of injury to the eyes of any person engaged in any such work from hot sand thrown off.

20. Work in the manufacture of wire rope where there is a reasonably foreseeable risk of injury to the eyes of any person engaged in the work from particles or fragments thrown off from flying ends of wire.

21. The operation of coiling wire, and operations connected therewith, where there is a reasonably foreseeable risk of injury to the eyes of any person engaged in any such work from the particles or fragments thrown off or from flying ends of wire.

22. The cutting of wire or metal strapping under tension, where there is a reasonably foreseeable risk of injury to the eyes of any person engaged in such work from flying ends of wire or flying ends of metal strapping.

23. Work in the manufacture of glass and in the processing of glass and the handling of cullet, where in any of the foregoing cases there is a reasonably foreseeable risk of injury to the eyes of any person engaged in the work from particles or fragments thrown off.

Part 2

Approved shields or approved fixed shields are required for:

24. Any process involving the use of an exposed electric arc or an exposed stream of arc plasma.

Part 3

Approved eye-protectors, shields or fixed shields must be supplied for the following specified processes:

25. The welding of metals by means of apparatus to which oxygen or any flammable gas or vapour is supplied under pressure.

26. The hot fettling of steel castings by means of a flux-injected burner or air carbon torch, and the de-seaming of metal.

27. The cutting, boring, cleaning, surface conditioning or spraying of material by means of apparatus (not being apparatus mechanically driven by compressed air) to which air, oxygen or any flammable gas or vapour is supplied under pressure excluding any such process elsewhere specified, where in any of the foregoing cases there is a foreseeable risk of injury to the eyes of any person engaged in the work from particles or fragments thrown off or from intense light or other radiation.

28. Any process involving the use of an instrument which produces light amplification by the stimulated emission of radiation, being a process in which there is a reasonably foreseeable risk of injury to the eyes of any person engaged in the process from radiation.

Part 4

Approved eye-protectors, approved shields or fixed shields must be supplied for the seven specified processes listed in this part:

29. Truing or dressing of an abrasive wheel where in either of the foregoing cases there is a reasonably foreseeable risk of injury to the eyes of any person engaged in the work from particles or fragments thrown off.

30. Work with drop hammers, power hammers, horizontal forging machines, and forging presses, other than hydraulic presses, used in any case for the manufacture of forgings.

31. The dry grinding of materials by applying them by hand to a wheel, disc or band which in any such case is power driven or by means of power-driven portable tool, where in any of the foregoing cases there is reasonably foreseeable risk of injury to the eyes of any person engaged in the work from particles or fragments thrown off.

32. The fettling of metal castings, involving the removal of metal, including runners, gates and risers, and the removal of any other material during the course of such fettling, where in any of the foregoing cases there is reasonably foreseeable risk of injury to the eyes of any person engaged in the work from particles or fragments thrown off.

33. The production of metal castings at pressure die casting machines, where there is a reasonably foreseeable risk of injury to the eyes of any person engaged in such work from molten metal thrown off.

34. The machining of metals, including any dry grinding process not elsewhere specified, where there is a reasonably foreseeable risk of injury to the eyes of any person engaged in such work from particles or fragments thrown off.

35. The welding of metals by an electric resistance process or a submerged electric arc, where there is a reasonably foreseeable risk of injury to the eyes of any person engaged in any such work from particles or fragments thrown off.

Schedule 2

This states that protection is required for people who are at risk from but actually not employed in five specified processes, namely:

1. The chipping of metal, and the chipping, knocking out, cutting out or cutting off of cold rivets, bolts, nuts, lugs, pins, collars, or similar articles from any structure or plant or from any part of any structure or plant, by means of a hammer, chisel, punch or similar hand tool, or by means of a power-driven portable tool where in any of the foregoing cases there is a reasonably foreseeable risk of injury to the eyes of any person not engaged in any such work from particles or fragments thrown off.

2. Any process involving the use of an exposed electric arc or an exposed stream of arc plamsa.

3. Work with drop hammers, power hammers, horizontal forging machines and forging presses other than hydraulic presses used in any case for the manufacture of forgings.

4. The fettling of metal castings, involving the removal of metal, including runners, gates and risers, and the removal of any other material during the course of such fettling, where in any of the foregoing cases there is a reasonably foreseeable risk of injury to the eyes of any person not engaged in any such work from particles or fragments thrown off.

5. Any process involving the use of an instrument which produces light amplification by the stimulated emission of radiation, where in any such process there is a reasonably foreseeable risk of injury to the eyes of any person not engaged in the process from radiation.

British standards for eye-protectors

There are various guidelines concerning the construction and marking, etc. of eye-protectors. The British Standards relating to the various types are:

BS 2092 (1987). *Eye-protection for industrial and non-industrial uses.*

BS 679 (1989). *Filters for use during welding and similar operations.*

BS 1542 (1982). *Equipment for eyes, face, and neck protection against non-ionizing radiation arising during welding and similar operations.*

BS 2724 (1987). *Specification for sun glare eye protectors for general use.*

BS 4110 (1970). *Eye-protection for vehicle users.*

BS 7028 (1988). *Guide for selection, care, and maintenance of eye protectors for industrial and other uses.*

BS 7192 (1989). *Specification for radiation safety of laser products.*

The British Standard of greatest interest to the optometric practitioner is BS 2092. This covers eye-protectors such as prescription safety spectacles.

BS 2092 (1987). Eye-protectors for industrial and non-industrial uses

Types of hazards against which eye-protection is required are:

(1) impact;
(2) molten metal;
(3) dust;
(4) gas;
(5) liquids;
(6) any combination of the above.

The eye-protectors include spectacles, goggles (box and cup types) and face shields (also known as face screens or visors).

Construction of eye-protectors

All eye-protectors should be constructed and designed to withstand the tests mentioned in Table 7.2.

The various tests can be summarized briefly as follows:

CONDITIONING TEST
The eye-protector is placed in an oven for 30 min at 55 °C ± 2 °C. It is then allowed to return to room temperature before carrying out further tests, such as robustness, optical quality, and impact resistance.

ROBUSTNESS TEST
The eye-protector must withstand a 6.35 mm steel ball striking the lens, and other parts, at 12 m/s.

Table 7.2 Schedules of tests for eye-protectors in BS 2092 (reproduced with kind permission of BSI)

Type of eye protection	Tests for all	Additional tests
Basic	Conditioning and	–
Impact	optical quality	Impact
Molten metal	Conditioning and	Molten metal and hot solids*
Liquid droplet	robustness	Liquid droplet
Liquid splash	Cleaning	Liquid splash*
Dust	Corrosion	Dust
Gas	Ignitability	Gas
Combination of above		As appropriate

* Liquid splash test must also be applied to molten metal eye-protectors if they are in the form of a face screen.

OPTICAL QUALITY

The accuracy and quality of the protective lenses is assessed. They should transmit at least 80 per cent of (visible) light, except when they are impact-resistant and are double layered, when the transmission should be at least 70 per cent. The lenses should be made of plastics material, of toughened or laminated glass, or of any combination of these materials. Untreated glass may be used only if it is backed with one of the foregoing materials.

IGNITABILITY TEST

A heated metal rod is placed in contact with the eye-protector to determine the ignitability index of the eye-protector.

CORROSION TEST

Metal parts of the protector are immersed in sodium chloride and then assessed for signs of corrosion. This is to eliminate the use of metals or alloys affected by perspiration.

CLEANING TEST

All eye-protectors should be capable of effective cleaning and show no signs of deterioration.

Satisfactory performance in the above tests allows the eye-protector to be classified as a basic type. The following additional tests must be carried out to allow the protector to be classified as giving protection against impact, molten metal, etc.

IMPACT RESISTANCE

The eye-protector must withstand a 6.35 mm steel ball striking it at 120 m/s for Grade 1 and at 45 m/s for Grade 2. Grade 1 lenses should be made of plastics material, except when double lenses are used. Grade 1 impact eye-protectors may only be goggles or face shields, not spectacles.

MOLTEN METAL AND HOT SOLIDS
Lenses must be resistant to the penetration of hot solids and the molten metal must not adhere to any part.

LIQUID DROPLET AND SPLASH, DUST, AND GAS TESTS
The eye-protectors are tested for resistance to the appropriate hazard. For the precise details of these test procedures see the appendix to standard 2092.

Lenses

Filters (tinted lenses) may be used in the various types of eye-protectors. Prescription spectacles may be made up for basic or impact resistance Grade 2. A manufacturer of prescription lenses must state the minimum substance of their lenses and samples of the lenses should be tested. Prescription lenses must also comply with the requirements of BS 2738 *Spectacle lenses*.

Side shields

Impact-resistant spectacles must provide lateral protection to the orbital cavities and must therefore be fitted with side shields Any spectacle claiming to be impact resistant should have side shields that at least meet the requirement of the robustness test. The side shields do not need to marked if they are as strong as the rest of the eye protector but, if they are only to 'robustness' strength, they must be marked BS 2092. Basic spectacles do not have to have side shields, but if they do, these must withstand the robustness test.

Marking of eye-protectors

Table 7.3 shows the required marking of eye-protectors. The eye-protector should also be accompanied by a description, in words, of the purpose for which it has been designed, i.e. type of eye-protector.

The kitemark is the registered mark of the British Standards Institution. For it to be used, a manufacturer must have a licence granted by the BSI. To obtain the licence, the quality control and products are surveyed by the BSI.

If the eye-protector has a kitemark the purchaser has the assurance that it conforms to the standard to which it claims to adhere. It is not mandatory for eye-protectors to be kitemarked but if there is no kitemark the purchaser must rely on the manufacturer's assurance.

Supply of prescription eye-protectors

Only companies that have accepted the requirements of The British Standards Institute (BSI) Quality Assessment Schedules are allowed to provide kitemarked prescription eye-protectors. This scheme allows companies to become registered if they can satisfy the high levels of quality control. Other firms may buy lenses from these BS 2092 licence holders without having to carry out the usual tests themselves.

Table 7.3 Marking of eye-protectors (BS 2092) (reproduced with kind permission of BSI)

Type of eye-protector	Lens marking*	Housing marking*
All eye-protectors	(1) BS 2092 (2) Manufacturer's mark or licence number	(1) BS 2092 (2) Manufacturer's mark or licence number
Liquid droplet	(1) BS 2092 (2) Manufacturer's mark or licence number	(1) BS 2092 (2) Manufacturer's mark or licence number (3) Letter 'C'
Liquid splash	(1) BS 2092 (2) Manufacturer's mark or licence number	(1) BS 2092 (2) Manufacturer's mark or licence number (3) Letter 'C'
Dust	(1) BS 2092 (2) Manufacturer's mark or licence number	(1) BS 2092 (2) Manufacturer's mark or licence number (3) Letter 'D'
Gas	(1) BS 2092 (2) Manufacturer's mark or licence number	(1) BS 2092 (2) Manufacturer's mark or licence number (3) Letter 'G'
Molten metal	(1) BS 2092 (2) Manufacturer's mark or licence number (3) Letter 'M'	(1) BS 2092 (2) Manufacturer's mark or licence number (3) Letter 'M'

Impact
  Grade 1
  Grade 2
	(1) BS 2092
	(2) Manufacturer's mark or licence number
	(3) Figure '1' or '2'
		(1) BS 2092
		(2) Manufacturer's mark or licence number
		(3) Figure '1' or '2'

Combination impact and/or molten metals with liquid splashes and liquid droplets, dusts or gases	(1) BS 2092 (2) Manufacturer's mark or licence number (3) Letter 'M' if appropriate (4) Figure '1' or '2' if appropriate	(1) BS 2092 (2) Manufacturer's mark or licence number (3) Letter 'C' 'D', 'G' or 'M' or figure '1' or '2' as appropriate

* Marking BS 2092 on or in relation to a product represents a manufacturer's declaration of conformity, i.e. a claim by or on behalf of the manufacturer that the product meets the requirements of the standard. The accuracy of the claim is therefore solely the responsibility of the person making the claim. Such a declaration is not to be confused with third party certification of conformity, which may also be desirable.

Protection against hazardous radiations

BS 1542 (1982) specifies the equipment necessary to protect the eyes, face, and neck against harmful radiations and incorporates protective filters conforming to the requirements of BS 679 (1989); these two standards should therefore be read in conjunction. Together they provide protection from glare, UV, and IR radiation.

Classification of protection requirements BS 1542

Class 1

Work, other than actual welding, but near welding operations, where some protection from harmful radiation is required but where good general vision is also necessary.
Recommended equipment: spectacles, goggles, face shields, hand shields, helmets, or fixed shields.

Class 2

Gas welding and cutting, which involves direct exposure to radiation of heat and light, sparks and particles of metal, and where moderate reduction of transmitted, UV, and visible radiation is necessary.
Recommended equipment: goggles, face shields, hand shields, helmets, or fixed shields.

Class 3

Electric-arc welding, cutting, and similar processes involving direct exposure to high intensity radiation, sparks, and particles of metal, together with risk of electric arcing from tools. This type of work requires a large reduction of the UV, IR and visible radiation.
Recommended equipment: face shields, hand shields, helmets or fixed shields. In some circumstances neck shields may also be necessary.

Class 4

Gas-shielded arc welding and cutting involving exposure to large amounts of UV, IR, and visible radiation both direct and reflected together with particles of metal ejected from the arc region.
Recommended equipment: helmets as for Class 3, but with provision for auxiliary heat-absorbing filter as recommended in BS 679. Neck shields may also be necessary.

The types of protective devices are:

(1) spectacles;
(2) goggles;
   (a) cup;
   (b) box;
(3) face shields;
(4) hand shields;
(5) neck shields;
(6) helmets;
(7) fixed shields.

All these types of protective devices are subjected to tests for robustness, corrosion, ignitability, and disinfection. The materials that come into contact with the skin must be of a type that is not known to cause irritation.

Hand shields and helmets are subjected to an additional, electrical insulation test.

The details of the gas and electric welding filters covered by BS 679, with recommendations as to their use, are given in Appendix C (see p. 208).

Marking filters

(1) gas welding without flux   GW
(2) gas welding with flux   GWF
(3) electric welding without flux   EW

The filters shall be permanently marked with the following details:

1. Manufacturer's name, trade mark, or licence number.

2. The figure denoting the shade number or, if a variable filter, the shade numbers in the light and dark states or, if a dual shade filter, the shade numbers of each zone.

3. The number of the British Standard, e.g. BS 679.

4. The letters denoting for which type of welding process they are suitable, i.e. GW, GWF, EW.

5. The letter 'R' if the filter is robust or 'NON-R' if the filter requires the addition of a backing lens to comply with the robustness requirements.

6. If appropriate, the impact grade as specified in BS 2092.

If protection is required from mechanical hazards as well as from radiation, then a BS 2092/1542 product is advisable. When welding with flux, the tint supplied must be darker, because the light given off is more intense. Gas welding emits less UV and IR radiation than electric welding, but protective filters are still required.

Selection of the appropriate eye-protector

Figure 7.1 can be used in the selection of an appropriate eye-protector.

European activities concerning eye-protection

There is now a European Committee for Standardization (CEN), which has a technical committee dealing with matters relating to eye-protection (CEN/TC58). Table 7.4 shows the current state of work on eye-protection. One of the standards has dual numbers—EN 165 has been published as a dual numbered British Standard, BS 6967. Other standards, EN 169, 170 and 171 have now been republished and have to be accepted as national standards either by publication of an identical text or by endorsement by April 1993. Conflicting national standards will have to be withdrawn. It should be noted that the transmittance requirements

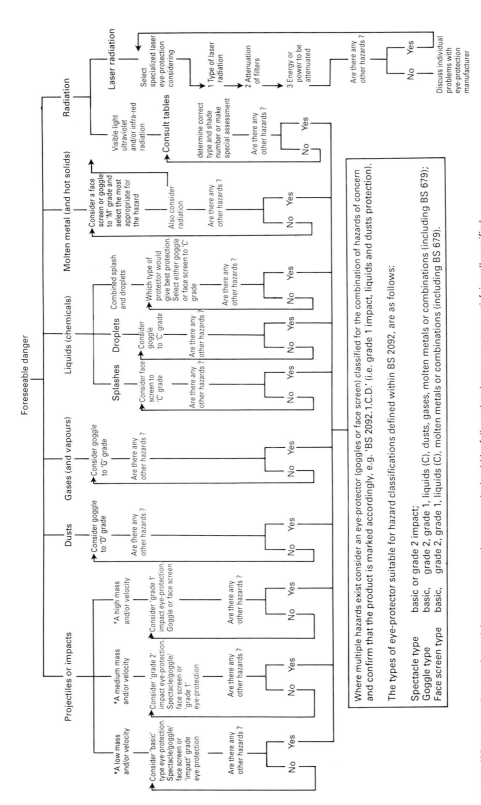

NOTE. Where more than one hazard, is present, more than one path should be followed and eye-protectors satisfying all specified conditions should be considered.

*The 'low' 'medium' and 'high' mass and/or velocity referred to above relate to the robustness and impact tests defined within BS 2092. As a guide to selection, the potential impact should be considered to be less than the test mass/velocity as follows:

Fig. 7.1 Flow chart for selecting appropriate eye-protectors from BS 7028 (reproduced with kind permission of BSI).

Table 7.4 European Standards for eye protection published and under development

CEN No.	Title	Status	Dual BS
EN 165	Personal eye-protection: vocabulary	Published April 1986	BS 6967
pr EN 166	Personal eye-protection: specifications	Awaiting formal vote	–
pr EN 167	Personal eye-protection: optical test methods	Awaiting formal vote	–
pr EN 168	Personal eye-protection: non-optical test methods	Awaiting formal vote	–
EN 169	Personal eye-protection: filters for welding and related techniques; transmittance requirements and recommended utilization	Published April 1986. Republished October 1992	No
EN 170	Personal eye-protection: ultraviolet filters; transmittance requirements and recommended utilization	Published April 1986. Republished October 1992	No
EN 171	Personal eye-protection: infra-red filters; transmittance requirements and recommended utilization	Published April 1986. Republished October 1992	No
pr EN 172	Personal eye-protection: Sunglare eye-protectors for industrial use	Circulated as prEN[†] May 1989	–
pr EN 207	Personal eye-protection: filters and eye protectors against laser radiation	Formal vote Aug 1992	–
pr EN 208	Personal eye-protection: eye-protectors for adjustment work on laser systems	Formal vote Aug 1992	–
pr EN 379	Welding filters with transmittance variable bytime and zone	Publication anticipated soon	–

[†] prEN is a draft standard circulated for comments.

of filters for welding in BS 679 (1989) agree with the appropriate requirements in EN 169.

EN 170 and EN 171 deal with filters for protection against ultraviolet and infra-red radiation. Filters should be marked with two numbers; the code number and the shade number. The transmittance requirements of the various filters are tabulated. Code numbers 2 and 3 are for fiilters to protect against ultraviolet and code number 4 is for protection against infra-red radiation. Table 7.5 shows some of the typical applications of the various filters when protection against ultraviolet is required. The selection of filters for protection against infra-red radiation is made according to the mean temperature of the source (in degrees Celsius). Copies of the European Standards are available from the BSI.

BS 2092: 1987 Specification for eye protectors for industrial and non-industrial uses is to be replaced by BS EN 166, 167 and 168. When a European Standard is introduced it will be prefixed by 'BS', so that EN

Table 7.5 Guidance for selection and use of filters to protect against ultraviolet radiation, EN 170 (1992) (reproduced by kind permission of BSI)

Scale number	Colour perception	Typical applications	Typical sources*
2–1.2	May be impaired	For use with sources which emit predominantly ultraviolet radiation and when glare is not an important factor	Low pressure mercury lamps such as lamps used to stimulate fluorescence or 'black lights'
2–1.4	May be impaired	For use with sources which emit predominantly ultraviolet radiation and when some definite absorption of visible radiation is required	Low pressure mercury lamps such as actinic lamps
3–1.2 3–1.4 3–1.7	No significant degradation	For use with sources which emit predominantly ultraviolet radiation at wavelengths shorter than 313 nm and when glare is not an important factor. This covers the UVC and most of the UVB bands[†]	Low pressure mercury lamps such as germicidal lamps
3–2.0 3–2.5	No significant degradation	For use with sources which emit intense radiation in both the UV and visible spectral regions and therefore require the attenuation of visible radiation	Medium pressure mercury lamps such as photochemical lamps
3–3 3–4			High pressure mercury lamps and metal halide lamps such as sun lamps for solaria
3–5			High and very high pressure mercury and xenon lamps such as sun lamps, solaria, pulsed lamp systems

* The examples given are for general guidance.
[†] The wavelengths of these bands are as recommended by CE (that is, 280 nm to 315 nm for UVB and 100 nm to 280 nm for UVC).

166 will become BS EN 166. Advice on the latest situation regarding standards can be obtained from the Enquiry Section, BSI, Milton Keynes MK14 6LE, telephone 0908 21166.

Acknowledgements

The extracts of Protection of Eyes Regulations are reproduced by kind permission of the Controller of Her Majesty's Stationery Office. The

British Standards are reproduced with kind permission of the BSI. Complete copies can be obtained by post from BSI Sales, Linford Wood, Milton Keynes, MK14 6LE; telex 825777 BSIMK G; telefax 0908 320856.

New regulations

Since this chapter was compiled there have been six new regulations introduced as amendments to the Health and Safety at Work etc. Act 1974. These are:

The Management of Health and Safety at Work Regulations 1992;

The Personal Protective Equipment Regulations 1992;

The Workplace (Health, Safety and Welfare) Regulations 1992;

The Provision and Use of Work Equipment Regulations 1992;

The Health and Safety (Display Screen Equipment) Regulations;

The Manual Handling Operations Regulations 1992;

The regulations of importance as far as eye protection is concerned are The Personal Protective Equipment Regulations 1992. For an outline of these new regulations see Appendix F. The above regulations are available from HMSO, mail order telephone 071 873 9090 or telefax 071 873 0011.

References

BS 679 (1989). *Filters, cover lenses and backing lenses for use during welding and similar operations.* BSI, London.

BS 1542 (1982). *Equipment for eye, face and neck protection against non-ionizing radiation arising during welding and similar operations.* BSI, London.

BS 2092 (1987). *Eye protection for industrial and non-industrial uses.* BSI, London.

BS 2724 (1987). *Specification for sun glare eye protectors for general use.* BSI, London.

BS 2738 (1985). *Tolerances on optical properties of mounted spectacle lenses.* BSI, London.

BS 4110 (1979). *Eye protectors for vehicle users.* BSI, London.

BS 7192 (1989). *Specification for radiation safety of laser products.* BSI, London.

BS 7028 (1988). *Selection, use and maintenance of eye-protection for industrial and other uses.* BSI, London.

Protection of Eyes Regulations. SI (1974). No. 1681, HMSO, London.

Protection of Eyes (Amendment) Regulations SI (1975). No. 303, HMSO, London.

Protection of Eyes Regulations Certificate of Approval Number 1. HMSO Publication No. F2475, HMSO, London.

Protection of Eyes Regulations Certificate of Approval Number 2. HMSO Publication No. F2489. HMSO, London.

Further reading

Rousell, D.F. (1979). *Eye protection.* ROSPA No. IS126. Royal Society for the Prevention of Accidents, Birmingham.

Taylor, S.P. and Austen, D.P. (1992). *Law and management in optometric practice,* (2nd edn). Butterworths-Heinemann, Oxford.

8. Lamps and lighting[*]

This chapter aims to outline the units of light, summarize the different types of light sources and luminaires, and describe lighting design procedures.

Concepts and units of light

Light is a form of radiant energy that induces a luminous sensation in the eye. The eye, as mentioned in Chapter 1, is more sensitive to some wave lengths than others, and this sensitivity is different for photopic and scotopic vision (Fig. 8.1). For photopic vision, the eye has a peak sensitivity at 555 nm, a yellow–green colour. For scotopic vision, the peak sensitivity shifts to 505 nm, a blue–green colour. There are, however, individual variations, and not everyone has the same sensitivity. To overcome this problem the CIE (Commission Internationale de l'Eclairage), an international lighting body, has adopted an agreed standard response, called the CIE standard observer. This is also known as the $v(\lambda)$ curve, which has maximum sensitivity under photopic conditions at 555 nm. At 400 nm the sensitivity is poor, being about one-thousandth of the maximum level. Therefore, 1 W of radiation of yellow–green colour will be 1000 times more effective than 1 W of radiation of a deep blue colour (Thorn Lighting 1991).

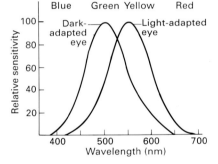

Fig 8.1 The relative spectral sensitivity of the human eye.

Photometric units

There are four important photometric units.

Luminous flux

The quantity of light emitted from a light source or received by a surface is expressed in units of lumens (lm). This is a measurement of the rate of flow of luminous energy, which is more commonly called the luminous flux. It is not practical to use the watt as a measure of light because of the variation in sensitivity of the eye with wavelength.

---

* The information in this chapter is mainly summarized from CIBS (1984), Pritchard (1985), EASL and LIF (1986), and Thorn Lighting (1991).

Illuminance

When a ray of light reaches a surface it is referred to as illumination. The quantity of illumination or illuminance (E) is defined as the luminous flux (F) that is incident on a given surface area (A), i.e. the luminous flux per unit area. This is expressed in SI units of lumens per square metre or lux (lx), where $E = F/A$. For example, if an area of 0.1 square metre receives a luminous flux of 40 lumens, the illuminance, E, will equal $40 \div 0.1$, i.e. 400 lux.

One of the basic laws to enable the calculation of illuminance is the Inverse Square Law, which states that the illuminance (E) equals the intensity of the light source (I) divided by the square of the distance (d); $E = I/d^2$. In principle this applies only to a point source of light in a completely black room. However, for most practical applications a luminaire can be considered to be a point source if its largest dimension is less than one-fifth of the distance from itself to the point of illumination. Therefore, the inverse square law can be applied to a 1-m fluorescent tube at a distance greater 5 m. For example, light from a small point source with a luminous flux of 1 lm, strikes a surface 1 m away, illuminating an area of 1 m^2. Hence, the illuminance $(E = F/A)$ is 1 lx. If the surface is moved to 2 m from the light source, the luminous flux will remain the same but the illuminated area will increase in size to 4 m^2, i.e. the area has increased in proportion to the square of the distance of the light source. The illuminance will be reduced to 0.25 lx, i.e. the illuminance has changed inversely with the square of the distance.

Luminous intensity

This is a measure of the capacity of a source or illuminated surface to emit light in a given direction. It is the luminous flux emitted in a very narrow cone containing the given direction divided by the solid angle of the cone. Luminous intensity (I) is expressed in candelas (cd). One candela is equal to one lumen per steradian; I = lm/sr (Fig. 8.2).

If a source emits the same luminous flux in all directions, its luminous intensity is uniform in all directions. However, for most sources the flux is not the same in all directions. A spotlight, for example, may have a luminous intensity of 2000 cd at the centre of the beam but, if it were angled, the intensity directed downwards may be reduced to only 200 cd. Applying the inverse square law to the spotlight when directed downwards on to a surface 2 m below, the illuminance will be:

$$E = I/d^2 \tag{8.1}$$

$$E = 2000/2^2$$

$$E = 500 \text{ lux}$$

where $I =$ intensity in candelas and $d =$ distance in metres. This law applies to light striking a surface at right angles. However, if the surface is tilted or turned so that the rays hit it at an angle, the illuminated surface will increase in size and the illuminance will decrease. The ratio of the originally illuminated area to the new area is equal to the cosine of the angle

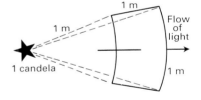

Fig 8.2 Luminous intensity. One lumen is the flow of light through an area of one square metre on a surface of a sphere of one metre radius with a point source of one candela at its centre (courtesy of EASL and LIF 1986).

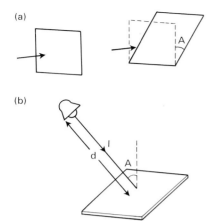

(a)

(b)

Fig 8.3 (a) The effect upon the illuminance of tilting a surface. (b) Inverse square law and the Cosine law (from the *Thorn Lighting Technical Handbook*, courtesy of Thorn Lighting Ltd).

through which the surface has been tilted. The illuminance will decrease by the factor of the cosine of the angle. This is known as the Cosine Law of Illuminance. For example, if a surface originally illuminated to 200 lx is tilted through an angle of 60 degrees, the illuminance will be reduced by half, to 100 lx, because the cosine of 60 degrees is 0.5 (Fig. 8.3(a)).

The Cosine Law can be combined with the Inverse Square Law, (Fig. 8.3(b)) thus:

$$E = \frac{I \; Cos \; A}{d^2} \qquad (8.2)$$

This equation can be used for one or more light sources provided the total illumiunance at a point is the sum of the illuminance by the individual sources; this is known as the point-by-point method.

Luminance

Luminance is the intensity of light emitted or reflected in a given direction per projected area of a luminous or reflecting surface. Luminance is expressed in candelas per square metre. For a matt surface the relationship is:

$$Luminance \; (cd/m^2) = \frac{Illuminance \; (lx) \times reflectance}{\pi} \qquad (8.3)$$

It should be noted that the terms 'luminance' and 'brightness' have similar meanings. However, the objectively measured photometric quantity should be referred to as luminance.

For physiological purposes the following approximate luminance ranges are recognized (i) scotopic conditions, 10^{-6} to 10^{-3} cd/m²; (ii) mesopic conditions, 10^{-3} to 3 cd/m²; and (iii) photopic conditions, 3 cd/m² upwards.

Contrast

This term is used subjectively and objectively. It expresses the luminance differences of two parts of the visual field. It may be expressed as:

$$Contrast = \frac{L - L1}{L} \qquad (8.4)$$

Where L is the task luminance and $L1$ is the background luminance.

Light sources

For the present purposes, there are two basic sources of light: (i) natural daylight; and (ii) electric (artifical) light.

Daylight

Although daylight appears to have a great advantage over electric light in being free of charge, it does have a major disadvantage in that it is a continually varying source. An electric light source is constant and, provided there is a supply of electricity, it is always available. Daylight, unfortunately, varies in quantity, colour, and direction depending upon the time of day, season, and weather conditions. For example, the range of illuminances can vary from 100 000 lx on a bright, sunny day to 5000 lx on an overcast day, and 0.5 lx from moonlight. To utilize the available daylight efficiently, large windows are required. These have several disadvantages, they:

(1) are poor thermal barriers;
(2) are poor noise barriers;
(3) require regular cleaning.

The spectral composition of daylight varies, as do the correlated colour temperatures (CCT) which can vary from 4000 K on an overcast day to 40 000 K on a clear, bright day; the most common value is about 6000 K. Five phases of CCT have therefore been agreed, which represent the typical spectral distribution of irradiances produced by the sun. As the CCT increases, i.e. with clear sky conditions, the blue end of the spectrum becomes more dominant. Correlated colour temperature is the temperature of a full radiator, which emits radiation having a chromaticity nearest to that of the light source being considered; it is measured in degrees Kelvin.

Electric light

To enable a comparison to be made between the different light sources the following factors can be assessed:

Luminous efficacy

The amount of light given by a lamp for each watt of energy consumed. It is measured in lumens/watt.

It is important to note that a discharge lamp can not normally be operated directly from mains electricity supply unless it has control gear to stabilize the lamp current. This control gear also consumes energy and, therefore, the efficiency of the discharge lamp circuit depends on the power taken by both lamp and control gear.

Colour properties

These are related to the spectral composition of the emission:

COLOUR RENDERING

This expression describes the appearance of colours under a given light source compared with their appearance under a reference source. Good colour rendering implies similarity of appearance under an acceptable light source, such as daylight. However, the colour appearance of light from a source is not a guide to its colour properties, as it is possible for the light from two lamps to be apparently identical in appearance but to have different colour rendering properties.

The CIE has developed a method of indicating the colour rendering properties of a light source. Table 8.1 shows the CIE general colour rendering index and Chartered Institute of Building Services (CIBS) Code classification. Accurate colour matching requires good colour rendering. Hence, light sources from Group 1A should be used. These have a high CIE general colour rendering index, being greater than or equal 90. The CIBS Code (1984) indicates the colour rendering group for the various types of light sources.

Table 8.1 Correlated colour temperature classes and colour rendering groups (from CIBS 1984 reproduced courtesy of the Chartered Institute of Building Services)

Correlated colour temperature (CCT)	CCT class	Colour rendering groups	CIE general colour rendering index (R_a)	Typical application
CCT ≤ 3300 K 3300 K < CCT ≤ 5300 K 5300 K < CCT	Warm Intermediate* Cold	1A	$R_a \geq 90$	Wherever accurate colour matching is required, e.g. colour printing inspection.
		1B	$80 \leq R_a < 90$	Wherever accurate colour judgements are necessary and/or good colour rendering is required for reasons of appearance, e.g. shops and other commercial premises.
		2	$60 \leq R_a < 80$	Wherever moderate colour rendering is required.
		3	$40 \leq R_a < 60$	Wherever colour rendering is of little significance but marked distortion of colour is unacceptable.
		4	$20 \leq R_a < 40$	Wherever colour rendering is of no importance at all and marked distortion of colour is acceptable.

* This class covers a large range of correlated colour temperatures. Experience in the UK suggests that light sources with correlated colour temperatures approaching the 5300 K end of the range will usually be considered to have a 'cool' colour appearance.

COLOUR APPEARANCE

The colour appearance is the colour the light source, or a white surface seen by its light, appears to be. It is generally described as being warm, intermediate, or cool. Cool colours have a blueish tinge, while warm colours are at the red end of the spectrum. Filament lamps have a warm appearance, whilst high pressure mercury lamps have a cool appearance. The colour of a light emitted by a near white source can be indicated by its correlated colour temperature (CCT). For example, the colour of a full radiator at 3500 K is the nearest match to that of a white tubular fluorescent lamp. Each lamp has its own specific CCT but, for practical purposes, these have been divided into three classes, as previously mentioned: warm, intermediate, and cold (Table 8.1).

Lamp life

The term 'life' of an electric lamp can have two different meanings:

1. The time after which the lamp ceases to operate, e.g. filament lamps fail due to filament breakage.
2. The time after which the light output is so reduced that it is more economical to replace the lamp, e.g. discharge lamps.

It is convenient to divide lamps into two main categories: (i) incandescent; and (ii) discharge lamps. These will be considered below. Most of the information was gathered from CIBS (1984), Pritchard (1985), Thorn Lighting (1991) and EASL and LIF (1986).

Incandescent lamps

Tungsten

Tungsten lamps operate by heating a tungsten filament to incandescence in a glass envelope filled with an inert gas, usually argon or krypton (Fig. 8.4). The passage of electricity through the filament raises the temperature of the tungsten molecules to the point where they emit light or incandesce. The resulting spectral emission is a function of the temperature of the filament. The main characteristic of the incandescent lamp is that the spectral emission forms a continuum (Fig. 8.5). As the temperature of the filament increases, the peak of its emission moves from the red to the blue end. Although the melting point of tungsten is 3600 K, the rate of evaporation increases markedly above 2800 K. This can be reduced by raising the vapour pressure in the lamp with a inert gas such as argon.

ADVANTAGES

(1) immediate full light output generally;
(2) operates in all positions;
(3) easy to control lamp output by varying applied voltage.

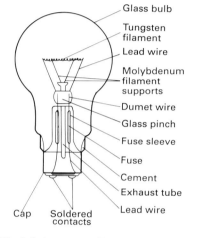

Fig 8.4 A tungsten filament lamp (from the *Thorn Lighting Technical Handbook*, courtesy of Thorn Lighting Ltd).

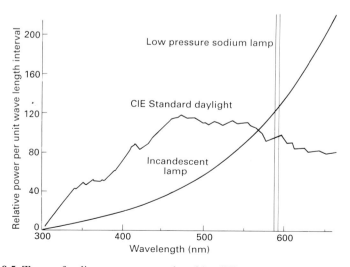

Fig 8.5 Types of radiant energy as produced by different light sources.

DISADVANTAGES

(1) short life (1000–2000 h), frequent replacement necessary;
(2) high running cost due to poor luminous efficiency (11–19 lm/W);
(3) emphasizes red strongly and yellows and greens to a lesser extent. Blue is strongly subdued;
(4) should not be used for colour matching;
(5) light output and life sensitive to small voltage variation;
(6) sensitive to vibrations;
(7) at too high a temperature the tungsten evaporates from the filament, leaving black deposits on the inside of the bulb, which reduce the light output.

Tungsten halogen

These are filament lamps. The filament is contained in a tube of fused silica or quartz, which is filled with a halogen compound gas.

Whereas conventional tungsten filament lamps must not be run at too high a temperature, a tungsten halide lamp can be run at much higher temperatures because, although the tungsten is evaporated off the filament, it combines with the halogen, e.g. iodine vapour, to form a reusable compound—a halide. This compound is carried on the convection currents within the bulb and, when it passes the filament, it dissociates into tungsten, which is deposited on the filament while the halogen is released to repeat the cycle (Fig. 8.6). This increases lamp efficacy and life.

ADVANTAGES

(1) higher luminous efficacy than tungsten (17–25 lm/W);
(2) longer life of lamp (2000–4000 h);
(3) no decline in light output with time (there is no blackening of the inner surface of the glass);
(4) higher colour temperature;
(5) lamps can be made small and compact, and therefore ideal for optometric instruments.

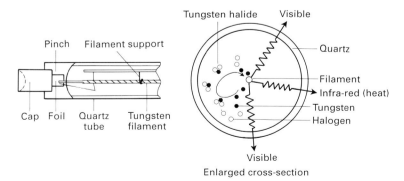

Fig 8.6 Simplified mechanism of the tungsten halogen lamp (from the *Thorn Lighting Technical Handbook*, courtesy of Thorn Lighting Ltd).

DISADVANTAGES
  (1) surface of bulb liable to deteriorate if touched with the fingers (the fats from the skin migrate into the quartz envelope, causing it to blister).

Gas discharge lamps

These lamps utilize the ionization of a gas to produce light. As electrons pass through the gas between the electrodes they accelerate and collide with the atoms of the gas (usually sodium or mercury). The collisions may cause: (i) ionization of the atoms, i.e. release an increasing number of free electrons, which themselves cause collisions, resulting in a cumulative ionization; or (ii) absorbtion by the gas atoms of most of the energy of the electrons, which raises the energy state of the electrons to higher levels. Subsequently, when the electron falls back to a lower energy level it emits radiation.

The spectral emissions from discharge lamps tend to be discontinuous, unlike those of incandescent lamps. At low gas pressure the emission is concentrated in narrow spectral lines, but these broaden as the pressure is raised.

The envelope of the lamp is filled with a mixture of gases and vapours. The main gas is the one responsible for the emission of light, i.e. mercury or sodium. Other gases are included to aid the starting of the electron discharge, such as argon, neon, xenon, or argon mixed with nitrogen. Control of the lamp current is achieved by either a large resistor or an inductive resistor, which is known as a choke or ballast. Virtually all discharge lamps require control gear of some sort. This will vary in size and weight in prortion to the lamp wattage and lamp complexity.

They are four main groups of discharge lamps:

  (1) low pressure;
  (2) high pressure;
  (3) sodium;
  (4) mercury.

Low pressure mercury lamps

These lamps are better known as tubular fluorescent lamps, or strip lights. This type of lamp produces radiation in the visible and UV regions, the latter being absorbed by a phosphor coating on the inside of the glass tube, which re-emits the radiation in the visible region (Fig. 8.7). Any UV radiation that is not absorbed by the phosphor is absorbed by the glass tube. The spectral emission can be varied by:

1. Varying the composition of the phosphors. There is a wide range of phospors available, which can produce almost any colour of light and different colour rendering properties. Phosphors commonly used are halophosphates, which produce 'white' light from a single phospor. Triphosphors, which use three phospors (red, green, and blue) in various combinations, give different shades of white, e.g. polylux and pluslux.

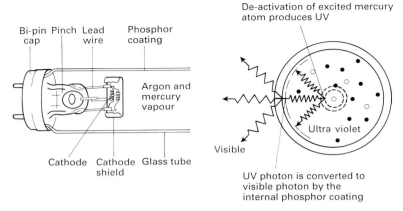

Fig 8.7 Simplified mechanism of a low pressure mercury vapour fluorescent lamp (from the *Thorn lighting handbook*, courtesy of Thorn Lighting Ltd).

The spectrum is a continuum (which varies with the phosphors used) on which the visible lines from the mercury discharge are superimposed.

2. Introducing an additional compound into the discharge tube, such as sodium, thallium or other metal halides. These improve both the colour properties and the light output.

Compact fluorescent lamps

These are smaller versions of the long discharge tube, in that they have been folded into a more compact form. For example, they may be folded into a D or L shape. They use approximately one-quarter the power of tungsten filament lamps and last, on average, five to ten times longer. They fall into two categories: (i) a replacement for general lighting systems (GLS) as an energy saving plug-in replacement; or (ii) light sources for new luminaires.

High pressure mercury discharge lamps

There are four types of high pressure mercury discharge tubes:

(1) mercury tungsten discharge;
(2) mercury discharge (fluorescent);
(3) metal halide;
(4) metal halide fluorescent.

Mercury tungsten discharge lamp

This type of lamp has an electrical discharge in a high pressure mercury vapour atmosphere contained in an arc tube with a tungsten filament heated to incandescence. This is surrounded by a glass envelope, which is lined with a fluorescent coating.

ADVANTAGES

1. It is the only type of high pressure mercury lamp that does not need control gear.

1. It has the lowest luminous efficacy of all high pressure mercury discharge lamps (10–26 lm/W).

2. Run-up period to 90 per cent full light output takes 4 min, with re-ignition after 10 min.

3. Sensitive to voltage variations and vibrations.

4. Restricted operating positions.

Mercury discharge (fluorescent) lamp

This has an electric discharge in a high pressure atmosphere contained in an arc tube within a glass tube envelope with fluorescent coating, such as magnesium fluorogerminate or yttrium. This type of lamp has similar run-up times and life expectancy as the mercury tungsten discharge lamp, but it has a greater luminous efficacy (35–50 lm/W). It can be operated in any position.

Metal halide and metal halide fluorescent lamps

These lamps have the same construction as the mercury discharge (fluorescent) lamp, except that the tube also contains a halogen substance, which: (i) increases the luminous efficacy of the lamp to 45–80 lm/W; and (ii) improves the colour appearance and colour rendering of the lamp.

Additional colour correction and efficacy is given to the metal halide fluorescent discharge lamp by adding a phosphor coating to the outer envelope. The life and run-up period is slightly longer for these tubes than for the other high pressure mercury discharge tubes.

High pressure mercury lamps are available in a large range of wattages and colours. They are smaller than low pressure mercury (fluorescent) lamps and have approximately the same life and range of luminous efficacy. They have a wide range of applications from factories to shops, offices, and for area floodlighting.

Low pressure sodium lamps

Radiation emitted from these lamps is monochromatic and has a characteristic yellow colour. The spectral emission is concentrated at 589 and 589.6 nm, which lies close to the peak of the photopic curve, i.e. maximum luminous efficiency of the eye (see Fig 8.5). These lamps have the highest luminous efficacy of all types (70–135 lm/W).

DISADVANTAGES

1. Full light emission is not available instantly, the run-up time to 90 per cent output takes from 6 to 12 min.

2. The light emitted is virtually monochromatic (yellow) and can therefore be used only where colour distortions are not important, e.g. for street lighting.

High pressure sodium lamps

These lamps emit a more continuous spectrum than the low pressure sodium lamps and therefore have better colour properties. They have a luminous efficacy of 65–100 lm/W and, although it is not as high as the low pressure lamp, it is being used increasingly in industry, for road lighting in cities, and for floodlighting, etc., where the better colour properties are considered worthwhile despite the lower luminous efficacy. It is also a smaller lamp and easier to handle. Full light emission is not available instantly as the lamp takes about 5 min to warm up. If switched off, there is an interval of about 10 min before the lamp will re-ignite, although special circuits can reduce this to about 1 min.

There are new high pressure sodium deluxe lamps, which have good colour rendering properties and which are designed primarily for interior lighting as an energy-saving alternative to other sources, e.g. SONDL-TA and SONDL-E (Thorn Lighting 1991). These lamps operate at higher pressure and temperature, which results in improved colour rendering properties. The main applications are for leisure centres, social areas, swimming pools, sports halls, and as uplighters in office areas where there are visual display units.

Problems with electric lighting

Two particular problems are associated with electric lights and, in particular, with fluorescent lights.

Flicker

Most lamps are supplied by alternating current (AC) at a frequency of 50 or 60 Hz. A 50 Hz supply has 50 cycles or reversals of direction of the current each second, so that there are 100 pulses of current per second. The light output does not generally follow the curve of the current and the output from each half cycle is overtaken by the output from the next half cycle before it has decayed significantly. The effect of a succession of half cycles gives a 'ripple' in the output, and hence the flicker is not significant. The absence of flicker in most light sources is due to their construction, e.g. in high pressure mercury lamps the contribution to the light output from the phosphors is marked and, as the phosphors have a long after-glow, this tends to smooth the light output. However, as the lamp ages, the flicker may be reduced to 50 Hz or less; this is usually most noticable as a flicker at the end of the tube. It is usually best to replace the tube if flickering occurs, but sometimes it can be alleviated by shielding the ends of the tube.

Stroboscopic effects

The oscillation of the light output from a lamp can produce a stroboscopic effect even when the oscillation flicker is not detectable. It can cause moving machinery, etc. to: (i) appear stationary; (ii) move more slowly than it actually is doing; or (iii) appear to reverse the actual direction of rotation (CIBS 1984). These effects occur in particular when all the lamps contributing to the illuminance are supplied by the same phase of the same supply.

The stroboscopic effects may be reduced by the following methods:

1. Light the moving object with a lamp fed from two different out-of-phase AC supplies, or from two different phases of the same 3-phase supply.

2. Operate the lamps from high frequency supplies. Electronic circuits operating at 32 KHz overcome the problem of flicker (Thorn Lighting 1990).

3. Select a lamp with low flicker characteristics, e.g. high and low pressue mercury discharge lamps, but avoid low pressure sodium lamps as they can give rise to flicker.

4. Use tungsten filament lamps fed from a direct current (DC) supply or a reduced AC supply.

Summary

There are numerous light sources to chose from. Table 8.2 gives a summary of the luminous efficacy, CCT and class, colour rendering characteristics, and uses of the main types of light sources available. The manufacturers' literature should be consulted for further details and current data.

Luminaires

Most light sources emit light in all directions, but this can be wasteful and cause visual discomfort. The function of most luminaires is (Thorn Lighting 1991):

1. To redistribute the light from the lamp in preferred directions with the minimum of loss.

2. To reduce glare from the source.

3. To be acceptable in appearance and, in some cases, make a definite contribution to the decor.

4. To provide support, protection, and electrical connection to the lamp.

Luminaires can take many different forms, but they all fulfil the above functions. Four methods of light control are commonly used (Fig. 8.8):

(1) obstruction;
(2) diffusion;
(3) refraction;
(4) reflection.

Obstruction

The lamp is surrounded by an opaque enclosure with a limited size aperture. An example of this type is a downlight in a refined metal tube with an open bottom.

Diffusion

The lamp is enclosed by a translucent material, which increases the apparent size of the light source. This will reduce the brightness of the source. Most diffusers also absorb light, as much as 60 per cent being lost. The diffusion is achieved by: (i) ribbing or stippling a specular reflector; (ii) providing a glass cover of diffusing material, such as acid-etched or sand-blasted glass; or (iii) translucent glass or a plastic filter.

Table 8.2 Light sources for general lighting (courtesy of J. Baker, Electricity Association Services Ltd)

Name or type	Efficacy range*	Approx. CCT (K)†	Colour rendering characteristics	Typical applications
Incandescent filament lamps				
GLS	11–19	2700	Accuracy quite good but blues dull and reds bright	Homes, hotels, restaurants shop display, anywhere that sparkle is required.
Tungsten halogen	17–25	3000–3200	As above, but blues brighter	Display and area lighting
Tubular fluorescent lamps (older T12 types)				
Artificial daylight	20–40	6500	Very good. BS 950 Part 1	Used for critical colour matching
Deluxe Natural	15–35	3600	Good. All colours bright but greens slightly yellow	Was widely used in food shops but low efficacy has led to its replacement
Northlight	20–40	6500	Good	Industrial colour matching
Deluxe Warm White	20–45	3000–3200	Good. Blues slightly dull	Blends well with filament lamps. Homes, hotels, etc.
Kolor-rite, Trucolour 37	20–45	4000 4200	Very good. Slight distortion to blues and greens	Were standard in hospital clinical areas. Museums, shops with special need.
Natural	30–40	4000–4200	Good. Slight distortion but all colours bright	Offices and shops. Compromise between efficacy and rendering
Daylight	45–65	4300	Fair. Emphasizes yellows, reds dull	Used where colour not important
Warm white, White	45–65	3000–3500	Poor. Yellows bright most other colours dull	General purpose. Too often used in the home with poor results
Tubular fluorescent lamps (modern T8 types)				
Various, e.g. Pluslux	50–80	3000 3500 4000	Generally good	High efficacy versions of older T12 types

Table 8.2 (*continued*)

Name or type	Efficacy range*	Approx. CCT (K)†	Colour rendering characteristics	Typical applications
Various, e.g. Polylux, Colour 83/84	55–90	3000 3500 4000	Very good. Some slight risk of metamerism	The modern high efficacy good colour rendering lamp
Compact, e.g. 2D, PL, SL, Lynx, etc.	40–55	2700–3500	Generally good. Most use T8 phosphors	Mainly used as replacements for filament lamps
High pressure discharge lamps				
Mercury fluorescent (MBF)	35–50	circa 4000	Not good. Some distortion of all colours	Mainly industrial. Cheap circuit
Metal halide (MBI/MBIF)	45–80	3000–4000	Good. Roughly equal to a Natural fluorescent lamp	Offices and shops with a crisp appearance
High pressure sodium (SON)	65–100	2000–2200	Poor. All colours distorted. Blues dull reds/yellows bright	Standard source for industry and city streetlighting
Deluxe high pressure sodium (SONDL)	50–80	2300	Fair. Roughly equal to a White fluorescent lamp	Offices, shops, leisure complexes (warm appearance)
Low pressure sodium (SOX)	70–135	Not applicable	None. Monochromatic output	Almost exclusively for street and security lighting

* A range is shown for efficacy to allow for differences between manufacturers and wattages.
† A range is shown for CCT (correlated colour temperature) to allow for differences between manufacturers. Because of continuous improvement in products, manufacturers should be consulted for the latest data.

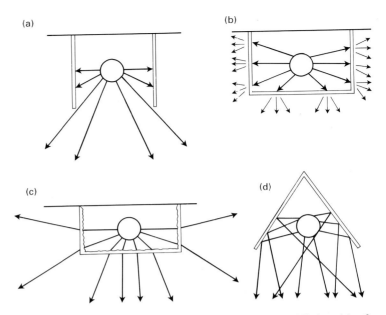

Fig 8.8 Four methods of light control. (a) Obstruction; (b) diffusion; (c) refraction; and (d) reflection (courtesy of the Electricity Association Services Ltd 1990—previously The Electricity Council).

Refraction

This technique uses numerous prisms to deviate the rays of light and redirect them in the direction required. The luminaire is generally made of glass or plastics and is highly suitable for general office lighting as it combines good glare control with reasonble efficiency.

Reflection

This technique makes use of reflecting surfaces, which may vary from a matt finish to a highly polished one. This type of luminaire is very efficient, as all the light can be directed where required. This is one of the oldest methods of controlling light and is seen in vehicle headlights, which have highly specular reflectors.

The methods described above are often combined in one luminaire. For example, a reflecting plate may be used above a lamp whilst prismatic controllers are used at the sides and below.

The British Standard that covers most of the luminaires in the UK is BS 4533 (1990). It is suitable for use with luminaires containing tungsten filaments and with tubular fluorescent and other discharge lamps running on supply voltages not exceeding 1 KV. The luminaires are classified according to: (i) type of protection against electric shock; (ii) degree of protection against ingress of dust or moisture; (iii) material of supporting surface for which luminaire is designed.

Luminaire characteristics can be listed as follows:

(1) mounting position;
(2) light distribution: polar curve shape, light output ratio, upward and downward light, British zonal system;
(3) spacing to height ratio;
(4) utilization factor;
(5) glare index.

Mounting position

Luminaires can be mounted in the following ways: (i) recessed into the ceiling; (ii) fixed on the ceiling (surface-mounted); (iii) suspended from the ceiling (pendant-mounted); (iv) free-standing; or (v) wall-mounted.

Polar curve shape

The distribution of light from a lamp or luminaire can be indicated graphically by a 'polar curve', which is the result of plotting the intensity of light in a series of directions within one vertical plane through the source. From the polar curve shown in Figure 8.9, it can be seen that the maximum intensity of light is vertically down, although there is some upward light.

In a symmetrical type of luminaire the polar curve will be virtually the same for all vertical planes. For example, filament lamps give a symmetrical distribution of light, and only one polar curve is required. Tubular fluorescent and other linear luminaires are known as non-symmetrical luminaires, as the distribution of light varies from one vertical plane to another. Most manufacturers therefore provide two polar curves for these non-symmetrical luminaires, one from the long axis and the other 90° to it, i.e. axial and transverse.

The polar curves can be used to calculate the total flux from a luminaire using the equation:

Light flux (lm) = intensity (cd) × solid angle (sr)   (8.5)

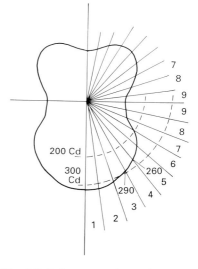

Fig 8.9 Polar curve (reproduced by courtesy of EASL and LIF 1986).

The intensity readings are taken at 10° intervals around the source. These intervals are described as 'zones', and the average intensity for each zone is then calculated. For example the average intensity for zone 4 shown in Figure 8.9 is:

$$\frac{290 + 260}{2} = 275 \, \text{candelas}$$

The plane angles must be converted to their equivalent solid angles, to obtain the 'zone factor'. Multiplication of the average intensity of each zone by the zone factor will give the total flux emitted from that zone. The zone factor will vary for each zone, being higher for zones nearer the horizontal than for those near the vertical (Table 8.3).

Hence, the total flux from zone 4 = 0.6828 × 275 = 172.5 lm

The sum of all the zone factors gives the total flux (in lumens) from the lamp or luminaire.

Table 8.3 Zone factors (courtesy EASL and LIF 1986)

Zone	Angle from vertical	Zone factor
1	0–10	0.095
2	10–20	0.284
3	20–30	0.463
4	30–40	0.628
5	40–50	0.774
6	50–60	0.897
7	60–70	0.993
8	70–80	1.058
9	80–90	1.091

Light output ratio

The ratio of the flux from the luminaire to that from the lamp is called the light output ratio (LOR):

$$LOR = \frac{\text{Light from luminaire}}{\text{Light from lamp}} \qquad (8.6)$$

$$\text{Upward/downward LOR} = \frac{\text{Upward/downward light from luminaire}}{\text{Light from lamp}} \qquad (8.7)$$

Upward and downward light

The proportion of the total light ouptut of the luminaire in the upper and lower hemispheres can be used to classify the luminaire. Luminaires providing most of their light downwards are called 'direct'; those whose light is mostly upwards are known as 'indirect', e.g. an uplighter. A general diffusing luminaire gives approximately equal amounts of light in all directions. The flux fraction ratio is the percentage of the total light from the luminaire in an upwards direction divided by the percentage of the total light from the luminaire in the downwards direction:

$$\text{Upper/lower flux fraction} = \frac{\text{Upward/downward light}}{\text{Total light from luminaire}} \qquad (8.8)$$

$$\text{Flux fraction ratio} = \frac{\text{Upper flux fraction}}{\text{Lower flux fraction}} \qquad (8.9)$$

Examples

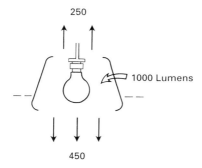

$$\text{LOR} = \frac{250 + 450}{1000} = 0.7 \text{ or } 70 \text{ per cent}$$

$$\text{Upward LOR} = \frac{250}{1000} = 0.25$$

$$\text{Downward LOR} = \frac{450}{1000} = 0.45$$

Upward LOR + Downward LOR = LOR

LOR = 0.25 + 0.45 = 0.7

$$\text{Upper flux fraction} = \frac{250}{250 + 450} = 35.71 \text{ per cent}$$

$$\text{Lower flux fraction} = \frac{450}{250 + 450} = 64.29 \text{ per cent}$$

Flux fraction ratio = 0.55

CIE Classification of luminaires

The CIE classification of luminaires is based upon the luminous flux directed above and below the horizontal (Table 8.4).

Table 8.4 CIE classification of luminaries

Luminaire	Flux above horizontal (%)	Flux below horizontal (%)
Direct	0–10	90–100
Semi-direct	10–40	69–90
General diffuse	40–60	40–60
Semi-indirect	60–90	10–40
Indirect	90–100	0–10

British zonal system

This is a method of classifying luminaires according to their downward light distribution as described in the CIBS Technical Memorandum No. 5. The polar curves are classified in terms of their nearest British Zonal (BZ) number, which range from BZ No. 1 to BZ No. 10. BZ No. 1 represents the maximum intensity when it is in the downward, vertical direction and BZ No. 10 when it is in the horizontal direction. It refers to the proportion of downward light that is directly incident on the working plane, in relation to the total flux emitted below the horizontal (the direct ratio). For any particular luminaire the direct ratio will increase with the room dimensions. It is possible to calculate the direct ratio for various sizes of rooms, if the polar curve is known, using the graph of direct ratio against room index (room size).

Space mounting to height ratio

Manufacturers' data accompanying luminaires should include the maximum spacing to height ratio. This defines the spacing of the luminaires (centre to centre) in relation to their height above the work surface, which is generally taken as being 0.85 m above the floor. This information should then allow the luminaires to be positioned so that they provide an even illumination on the work surface. The luminaires that are placed too far apart, will create some poorly lit areas.

If information is not provided by the manufacturer, the guide lines given in Table 8.5 may be used.

Utilization factor (coefficient of utilization)

The utilization factor (UF) gives a measure of the efficiency of the lamp/luminaire in providing uniform lighting in a room. The UF is the luminous flux that reaches the work surface directly, or by reflection, expressed as a ratio of the total luminous flux emitted from the lamp. The UF value will vary according to the size of room, the reflectances of the surfaces in the room, and the distribution and spacing of the luminaires. An indication of the range of UFs likely to occur in rooms of different sizes, with high and low surface reflectances, is given in the CIBS Code (1984) for different types of luminaires. These tables are calculated using the BZ system described in CIBS Technical Memorandum No. 5. Reference can

Table 8.5 Spacing:height ratio guidelines

BZ number	Maximum spacing : height ratio
1, 2	1.00 : 1.00
3, 4	1.25 : 1.00
5–10	1.50 : 1.00

also be made to the manufacturer's data, which frequently includes UFs for standard conditions.

UF × luminous efficacy of the lamp circuit
= installed efficacy of the installation

This is a measure of how much luminous flux reaches the working plane for each watt of energy applied. Luminaires can be ranked in order of installed efficacy and, therefore, the most efficient luminaire can be selected.

Glare index

The glare index system produces a numerical index calculated according to CIBS Technical Memorandum No. 10. It ranks the discomfort glare from lighting installations in order of severity and gives the permissible limit of discomfort glare from an installation quantitatively. The luminous intensity distribution from a luminaire and its projected area are important factors in calculating the glare index. Other factors are room dimensions, surface reflectances, and the position of the luminaires in relation to the line of sight. The CIBS Code (1984) gives an indication of the glare indices for square rooms of different areas with high and low reflectances for a regular array of various types of luminaires.

The BZ classification is being replaced by UF and Glare Index tables based on the calculation methods in CIBS Technical Memoranda Nos. 5 and 10.

Lighting design

So far, this chapter has discussed the different types of light sources and luminaires, i.e. how light is produced and its distribution. Now we need to discuss where and for what reason lighting is required. It can be used for several purposes:

1. To aid and facilitate the performance of a visual task.
2. To create an appropriate visual environment, i.e. aesthetic appearance.
3. To ensure safety of people.
4. To provide security for premises.

Lighting during the day can be provided by daylight, electric light, or a combination of both. People usually prefer to work in daylight and dislike being in rooms with no windows. However, windows can create uncomfortably hot conditions when there is plenty of sunlight and may also act as sources of glare. The most common approach to interior lighting is therefore to use both daylight and artificial light sources together, to produce the required task lighting; the artificial light acts as a supplement to daylight when and where it is insufficient.

Daylight

The extent to which daylight is available at a point inside a room is normally expressed as the 'daylight factor'. This is the illuminance received at a point on a plane in an interior from a sky of known or assumed luminance distribution, expressed as a percentage of the horizontal illuminance outdoors from an unobstructed hemisphere of the same sky (CIBS 1984). It is calculated in a similar method to the lumen design method (see p. 148). It takes into account the effect of windows and the amount of daylight they transmit, and this is divided by the total surface area of the room and a factor to allow for reflectances from the surfaces and windows.

When the average daylight factor is 5 per cent or more, the interior will appear to be well lit, and it should be sufficient for most of the day. If the average daylight factor is between 2 and 5 per cent then it may be worthwhile to consider using artificial light in addition to the available daylight. So when the daylight falls below the expected value the supplementary lighting can be used. For values of less than 2 per cent the interior will be poorly lit and artificial light sources will be required nearly all the time.

Artificial lighting

There are several methods by which a task may be illuminated. The three most common in use are shown in Figure 8.10 (CIBS 1984) and are referred to as:

(1) generalized lighting;
(2) localized lighting;
(3) local lighting.

General lighting system

These are lighting systems designed to provide an appropriate uniform illuminance over the entire working area. This has the advantage of allowing flexibility of work stations, as there is even illumination over the working area. However, energy is wasted because the whole area is illuminated to a level needed for the most critical task. It is therefore more costly than it need be. The luminaires are generally arranged in a regular layout, which is easy to plan using the lumen method of lighting design. It is recommended that the uniformity of illuminance over the task area should be not less than 0.8 (ratio of minimum luminance to average luminance; CIBS 1984).

Localized lighting

This system is designed to provide the required illuminance on the working surface, together with a lower level of illuminance for other general areas. The difference in illuminance between the task and general areas should be in the ratio of 3 : 1 or less (CIBS 1984). Great care must be taken at the design stage of this system to match the lighting to the work stations. If at a later date, the work stations are relocated, there may be a problem with fixed luminaires. This can be overcome if uplighters (stand- or desk-mounted) are used, as they can easily be moved to a new location.

Localized lighting will generally use less energy but may require more maintenance than generalized systems.

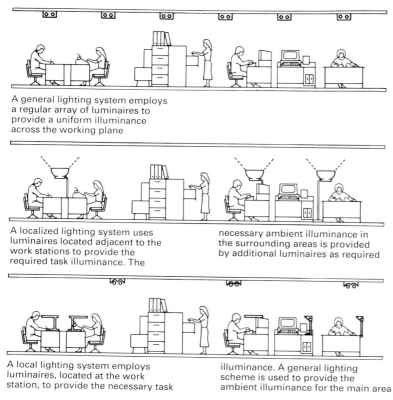

A general lighting system employs
a regular array of luminaires to
provide a uniform illuminance
across the working plane

A localized lighting system uses
luminaires located adjacent to the
work stations to provide the
required task illuminance. The

necessary ambient illuminance in
the surrounding areas is provided
by additional luminaires as required

A local lighting system employs
luminaires, located at the work
station, to provide the necessary task

illuminance. A general lighting
scheme is used to provide the
ambient illuminance for the main area

Fig 8.10 Lighting systems. (a) General; (b) localized; and (c) local (from CIBS 1984, reproduced courtesy of The Chartered Institute of Building Services).

Local lighting

This has two separate lighting systems: one to provide the ambient background lighting and the other to provide supplementary lighting at the task. Local lighting is a very efficient method of providing high task illuminance which can be flexible, directional lighting for detailed tasks. It is also a method whereby additional lighting can be provided at the task, the luminaire usually being mounted at the work station. Care must be taken when positioning the luminaire at the work station so that it does not create veiling reflectances or shadows, or become a glare source for the surrounding workers. Local light should not be placed directly in front of the worker as it will reduce the visibility. The best position is to the left of the work station or desk if the worker is right-handed, so that the reflections will mainly go across the worker's line of sight. For left-handed workers the local light should be positioned to the right. The task to background illuminance ratio should not be less than 3 : 1 (CIBS 1984).

This system has the advantage of providing the necessary level of lighting. But, unfortunately, the luminaires may be inefficient, rather expensive, and have higher maintenance costs due to increased wear and tear.

Lumen method of lighting design

This is a method of lighting design that will provide uniform illumination of an area when the luminaires are arranged in a regular layout. If the lighting is to vary over the working area then the point-by-point method should be used (see p. 128). The lumen method can be used to calculate the average illumination produced by a lighting installation, or the number of luminaires required to achieve the desired illuminance. The light received on a work surface will depend on the direct light and the reflected light. Therefore, when calculating the lighting to be installed to give a certain level of illuminance on the work surface, factors such as room size, reflectance of the surfaces, and type of lamp have to be taken into account. The number of luminaires (N) may be calculated from the equation (CIBS 1984):

$$N = \frac{E \times A}{F \times n \times \text{LLF} \times \text{UF}} \tag{8.10}$$

Where A = area of the work surface (m^2), E = average illuminance on the working surface (lux), F = lamp luminous flux (lumens), LLF = the light loss factor, n = the number of lamps per luminaire, and UF = the utilization factor.

Illuminance (E)

The CIBS Code (1984) recommends levels of illumination for many tasks and occupations. It may be consulted to determine the value of E that should be provided for a specific task.

Utilization factor (UF)

This information may be published by the manufacturers for standard conditions of use of their luminaires, or it may be calculated as described in CIBS Technical Memorandum No. 5. To use the UF tables correctly it is necessary to know the room size (room index) and the room reflectances of the ceiling, walls, and floor.

Light Loss Factor

The decreased light output from an installation due to dirt and ageing must be taken into account in lighting design. The light loss factor (LLF) is the ratio of illuminance produced by a lighting installation at some specific time compared to the illuminance produced when it was new.

$$\text{LLF} = \text{LLMF} \times \text{LMF} \times \text{RSMF} \tag{8.11}$$

Where LLMF, lamp luminance maintenance factor; LMF, luminaire maintenance factor; and RSMF, room surface maintenance factor.

LLMF is the proportion of initial light output that is produced after a specified time. The light output will decrease with time for most lamps, but the extent varies for the different types of lamp. The manufacturers' data should be consulted for the LLMF value for a specific number of hours for each lamp.

LMF takes into account the reduced light output that will occur due to dust and dirt being deposited on the luminaire. This can be calculated from tables and graphs in CIBS Code (1984) Appendix 7.

RSMF takes into account the altered reflectance that will occur as surfaces collect dust and dirt, which will in turn alter the illuminance produced by the lighting installation. The reduction of reflected light will have less effect if the luminaires have a strong downwards distribution. Note that indirect lighting, which is dependent upon reflections, will have a far greater reduction of light reaching the work surface. This can also be calculated from graphs in the CIBS Code (1984) Appendix 7.

The LLF has replaced a previous maintenance factor, which gave only one estimate of the illuminance that would be provided by the installation. The LLF allows an estimate of the illuminance at any specified time and so changes in illuminance with respect to time, can be assessed.

Recommended levels of illuminance

In the UK, statutory instruments such as the Health and Safety at Work Act (1974) and the Factories Act (1961) require lighting at places of work should be sufficient and suitable. This is normally taken to mean that the lighting on the tasks and in the areas where people circulate is adequate. The illuminance required for a particular task will depend on many factors, including the size of the detail, the contrast of the detail with its background, the accuracy and speed with which the task must be performed, the age of the worker, etc. Fortunately, recommendations that take these factors into account are given in the CIBS Code for Interior Lighting (CIBS 1984), which provides levels of illuminance for a variety of tasks and occupations. The Code gives a scale of standard service illuminance, which increases as the visual task becomes more difficult (Table 8.6). These standard service illuminance values assume that the task and/or interior is representative of its type in details, duration, etc. However, it can be modified if the task concerned differs from the assumed typical circumstances. Modifying factors can include visual difficulty, duration of the work, the prevalence of visual impairment (e.g. from scratched safety spectacles), and the consequence of any mistakes. A flow chart permits these modifying factors to be taken into account so that the standard service illumination can be modified to give a value known as the design service illuminance (Table 8.7). If the design service illuminance is 1500 lx or greater, it is recommended that local lighting should be considered along with the optical aids, e.g. magnifiers.

A good lighting system must provide suitable lighting for all employees, whatever their task and whatever their age. Older employees require higher levels of illuminance to achieve the same levels of visual efficiency. Therefore the level of illumination may need to be increased; this is most easily achieved by the use of local lighting. Care must be taken to ensure that this additional lighting does not become a glare source to other employees working in the surrounding area. Older individuals are more sensitive to glare than the young, due to increased light scattering within the eye, and also take longer to adapt from one lighting level to another.

Table 8.6 Examples of activities/interiors appropriate for each standard service illuminance (from CIBS 1984, reproduced courtesy of the Chartered Institute of Building Services)

Standard service illuminance (lx)	Characteristics of the activity/interior	Representative activities/interiors
50	Interiors visited rarely with visual tasks confined to movement and casual seeing without perception of detail	Cable tunnels, indoor storage tanks, walkways
100	Interiors visited occasionally with visual tasks confined to movement and casual seeing calling for ony limited perception of detail	Corridors, changing rooms, bulk stores
150	Interiors visited occasionally with visual tasks requiring some perception of detail or involving some risk to people, plant or product	Loading bays, medical stores, switchrooms
200	Continuously occupied interiors, visual tasks not requiring any perception or detail	Monitoring automatic processes in manufacture, casting concrete, turbine halls
300	Continuously occupied interiors, visual tasks moderately easy, i.e. large details > 10 min arc and/or high contrast	Packing goods, rough core making in foundries, rough sawing
500	Visual tasks moderately difficult, i.e. details to be seen are of moderate size (5–10 min arc) and may be of low contrast. Also colour judgement may be required	General offices, engine assembly, painting and spraying
750	Visual tasks difficult, i.e. details to be seen are small (3–5 min arc) and of low contrast, also good colour judgements may be required	Drawing offices, ceramic decoration, meat inspection
1000	Visual tasks very difficult, i.e. details to be seen are very small (2–3 min arc) and can be of very low contrast. Also accurate colour judgements may be required.	Electronic component assembly, gauge and tool rooms, retouching paintwork
1500	Visual tasks extremely difficult, i.e. details to be seen extremely small (1–2 min arc) and of low contrast. Visual aids may be of advantage	Inspection of graphic reproduction, hand tailoring, fine die sinking
2000	Visual tasks exceptionally difficult, i.e. details to be seen exceptionally small (< 1 min arc) with very low contrasts. Visual aids will be of advantage	Assembly of minute mechanisms, finished fabric inspection

Table 8.7 Flow chart for obtaining the design service illuminance from the standard service illuminance (from CIBS 1984, reproduced courtesy of the Chartered Institute of Building Services)

Standard service Illuminance (lx)	Are the task details unusually difficult to see?*	Are the task details unusually easy to see?*†	Is the task done for an unusually long time?*	Is the task done for an unusually short time?*†	Is visual impairment widespread among those doing the work?‡	Do errors have unusually serious consequences to people, plant or product?	Design Service Illuminance (lx)§‖
50	no / yes	50	50	no / yes	50	no / yes	50	no / yes	50	no / yes	50
100	no / yes	no	100	100	no / yes	100	no / yes	100	no / yes	100	no / yes	100
150	no / yes	150	150	no / yes	150	no / yes	150	no / yes	150	no / yes	150
200	no / yes	200	200	no / yes	200	no / yes	200	no / yes	200	no / yes	200
300	no / yes	300	300	no / yes	300	no / yes	300	no / yes	300	no / yes	300
500	no / yes	500	500	no / yes	500	no / yes	500	no / yes	500	no / yes	500
750	no / yes	750	750	no / yes	750	no / yes	750	no / yes	750	no / yes	750
1000	no / yes	1000	1000	no / yes	1000	no / yes	1000	no / yes	1000	no / yes	1000
1500	no / yes	1500	1500	no / yes	1500	no / yes	1500	no / yes	1500	no / yes	1500
2000	2000	no	2000	2000	no	2000	2000	2000

* The standard service illuminances recommended in the schedule are based on tasks which are representative of their type in the detail that has to be seen and the time for which the task has to be done. These steps in the flow chart allow for departures from these assumed conditions.

† The standard service illuminance of 200 lx is provided as an amenity for continuously occupied interiors, even when perception of task detail is not required.

‡ If the cause of visual impairment is dirty or scracthed spectacles, safety glasses, safety screens. etc., it may be more effective to clean or replace these items rather than change the lighting. If safety screens are acting as a source of veiling reflections then the lighting task worker geometry should be re–arranged.

§ If the design service illuminance is more than two steps on the illuminance scale above the standard service illuminance, consideration should be given to whether changes in the task details, the organisation of the work or the people doing the work are more appropriate than changing the lighting.

‖ For a design service illuminance of 1500 lx or 2000 lx, local lighting supplemented by optical aids should be considered.

These points should be remembered, particularly if there any complaints about the lighting system from older employees.

Of particular interest to ophthalmologists and optometrists is the CIBS (1989) guide, which recommends service illuminance levels:

Ophthalmology

Test room (working plane)	50–300 lx
Consulting room (working plane)	300 lx
Vision chart (vertical plane)	300 lx
Bjerrum screen	100 lx (maximum)
Chair (local)	1000 lx

Operating theatre

Operating cavity	10 000–50 000 lx

When Ishihara charts are used it is recommended that the colour temperature of the light source should be as near as possible to 6500 K.

The test rooms require black-out facilities and a means of dimming the general lighting.

Glare and its control

A good lighting system, as well as providing a suitable level of illumination, must avoid glare. There are two types of glare: disability glare, and discomfort glare.

Disability glare
The term 'glare' is usually thought of as the prescence of a very bright light source, such as car headlights or the sun, which prevents us from seeing the necessary detail. This type of glare is known as disability glare, which impairs the ability to see the detail without neccessarily causing visual discomfort. It is nearly always associated with excessive light received by the eye, either direct from the light source or by reflection from bright shiny surfaces.

Discomfort glare
This is defined as glare that causes visual discomfort without necessarily impairing the ability to see detail. It is therefore a less obvious type of glare and manifests itself in the form of discomfort.

Lighting systems in most interiors are more likely to cause visual discomfort than disability. The discomfort may not be apparent but its effects are cumulative and contribute to a sense of tiredness, especially towards the end of the day. People with poor health are particularly sensitive to visual discomfort caused by glare, as are elderly people. Discomfort glare (g) from a light source can be expressed (Electricity Council 1990):

$$g = \frac{B_S^{1.6} \times W^{0.8}}{B_B \times P^{1.6}} \times 0.478 \qquad (8.11)$$

Where B_S, luminance of source (cd/m^2); B_B, luminance of background (cd/m^2); W, angular size of source; and P, position index, which indicates the effect of position of source on the eye.

The CIBS Code (1984) also gives recommendations for the limiting glare index for the various tasks, etc. The limiting glare index specifies the degree of discomfort glare that is permissible from an overhead lighting installation (it is not applicable to local lighting installations). Calculation of the glare index is outlined in the CIBS Technical Memorandum No. 10 and the value calculated should not exceed the limiting values suggested. The values of the limiting glare index usually lie in the range of 10 (low glare) to 30 (high glare). For example, the limiting glare index advised for general offices is 19, whereas for warehouse storage areas it is 25.

Control of glare

It is often possible to reduce or avoid glare by:

1. The reflection factor of the object and the immediate background should be adjusted so that the contrast is adequate for seeing the task without being so high as to cause discomfort.
2. Where local lighting is provided the surrounding general illuminance should not fall to low, i.e. increase the background illuminance to reduce glare effects. The areas surrounding the task should be illuminated to not less than one-third of the task illuminance. Figure 8.11 shows the recommended illuminance ratios and surface reflectances (CIBS 1984).
3. Shiny or specular surfaces should be avoided where there is the possibility of bright images being reflected; use matt surfaces.
4. Luminaires should be installed at correct mounting heights and spacing, otherwise uneven lighting will occur.
5. Source luminance should be kept at a minimum; use diffusers or screens.
6. The solid angle subtended by the source at the observer's eye must be kept at a minimum.
7. Move the glare source out of the line of sight (i.e. increase P). This is easy if the lamps are suspended.
8. Visual tasks should not be located so that a window is near the line of sight. If this cannot be avoided the window should be screened to reduce its brightness.

The most common cause of glare from lighting installations is due to the direct view of bare fluorescent tubes or incandescent lights from the normal viewing angle. Uplighters are being used increasingly because they avoid glare by giving diffuse light. They are luminaires that direct most of the light upwards on to the ceiling or upper walls to illuminate the working plane by reflection.

Several different types of light source are used in uplighters. The two most common sources are the incandescent tungsten halogen and the high pressure sodium deluxe discharge lamps. Most uplighters have a

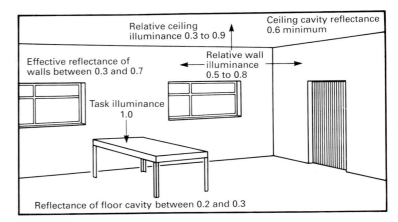

Fig 8.11 Recommended illuminance ratios and surface reflectances, (from CIBS 1984, reproduced by courtesy of The Chartered Institute of Building Services).

wide symmetrical light distribution (although this is reduced if they are wall mounted).

Choice of lighting equipment

Light Source

Once the lighting system has been designed, a list of suitable lamps should be made. The suitability of the lamp will depend on the nature of the task in the work place. Lamp selection should be based on the following factors (CIBS 1984):

1. Is good colour rendering required–either for accurate performance of the task or the aesthetic appearance of the area being illuminated?
2. Does the task require rapid provision of lighting? If the answer is yes, then most discharge lamps should be avoided as they need a run up time.
3. Lamp life and luminous efficiency must be considered. If luminaires are difficult to access then lamps requiring regular maintenance will be inappropriate.
4. Stroboscopic effects should be avoided if the work place has moving machinery.
5. The degree and accuracy of light control required for the task must be assessed. It is easier to control light from a small compact light source than a large one. The type of luminaires available must also be taken into account.

Luminaire

The following factors must be assessed regarding the work place and the specific task before a luminaire can be selected:

1. *Environmental conditions.* Does the luminaire have to withstand vibration, moisture, dust, and extremes of temperature? Such factors must

be taken into consideration—the luminaire must operate safely in the environmental conditions of the work place. The safety of the luminaire can be guaranteed by using equipment conforming to BS 4533 (1990), which covers the electric, mechanical, and thermal aspects of safety. The luminaires are classified according to the type of protection against electric shock, the degree of protection against dust and moisture (Ingress Protection (IP) System) and according to material of the supporting surface for which the luminaire is designed.

2. *Light distribution of luminaires.* This will influence the distribution of the light and the directional effects that will be achieved. The illuminance ratio charts of the CIBS Technical memorandum No. 15 can be used to assess the distribution of lighting and directional effects for a regular array of given luminaires. Illuminance ratio charts enable the effects of room size, reflectances of the surfaces, the luminaire direct ratio, and flux fraction ratios to be assessed. The most useful way to use the charts is to identify the range of reflectances and luminaires necessary to provide the recommended conditions. Each chart is marked with the direct ratio (expressed as the BZ number) along the horizontal axis and the flux fraction ratio along the vertical axis, while the recommended ranges are shown as 'safe areas'. This allows the range of acceptable luminaires to be selected according to their BZ number and flux fraction ratio.

3. *The utilization factor.* The UF of the luminaire and the luminous efficacy of the lamp will allow the efficacy of the installation to be calculated. This is a measure of the amount of luminous flux that reaches the work plane for each watt of power supplied. The luminaires all ranked according to the installed efficacy, so the most efficient may be chosen.

4. *Other factors.* Luminaire life, reliability, and the ease of maintenance should also be considered.

Lighting system management

The management must control the chosen lighting system so that it operates as efficiently as possible; it must also be maintained. Lights are often switched on in the morning and left on until the end of the work. This can be wasteful, as it may not be necessary for all the luminaires to be in use all the time. For example, luminaires near the windows can be switched off when daylight is adequate for the task and local lighting can be switched off when the work station is not being used. There are three methods by which lighting systems may be controlled (CIBS 1984; Electricity Council 1990):

(1) manual;
(2) automatic;
(3) processor control.

Manual control

The manual control of the lighting system, for example by a foreman, may appear to be a cheap method of control, although this is not always the case. The lights will be switched on when the daylight is inadequate, but are less likely to be switched off when the daylight becomes sufficient.

The control panels for work areas must be clearly marked so it is clear which switch controls which bank of lights or individual lights. It must be easily accessible and located in a convenient place.

Automatic control

This may be provided by photocells, which can monitor the level of useful daylight. These can either be of the type that simply switch on or off at preset levels, or they may increase or decrease the electric light, so that a certain level of illumination is maintained. The photo-electric type of control, which simply switches on or off, may control the whole working area or control only the lighting near to the windows. To prevent the lights from switching on and off because of passing clouds, they are usually fitted with a time delay. If dimming control is wanted then it should be noted that this may be used only with filament or tubular fluorescent lamps (Electricity Council 1990). This system is generally preferred by employees, as the light increases or decreases slowly—there is no sudden switching on or off. Time switches may also be used to switch lights on at the start of the day and, most importantly, off at the end of the day. All too often lights are left on overnight—a waste of money and energy. A manual over-ride should be available, so that unexpected circumstances can be dealt with, such as maintenance or cleaning outside of normal hours. Other control devices can detect the presence of a person within an area and switch on the lights. These will then be turned off after the area has been vacated for a set time. These devices include audio, ultrasonic and IR sensitive systems.

Processor control

These systems, which are either computer- or microprocessor-based, are becoming more popular. They can not only control lighting, but also building services, such as air-conditioning, fire alarms, and lifts. The great advantage of this system is its flexibility, in that the computer control programme can be adjusted to suit the work areas, and can be modified as required. The system can monitor the building continuously, so that it is operating at maximum efficiency and economy (CIBS 1984).

Measurement of illuminance and luminance

The most common measurement required is the level of illuminance, i.e. the amount of light falling on a surface. The CIBS Code (1984) and other lighting codes give recommended levels of illuminance (in lux) for various occupations and tasks; hence a method of measurement is required to check whether the level is appropriate. An illuminance meter usually consists of a light-sensitive cell, which is connected by an amplifier to a display; the display may be analogue or digital. The light-sensitive cell may consist of a selenium or silicon photo-voltaic cell, although neither of these have a spectral response similar to that of the human visual system. One method of matching the spectral sensitivity of the cell to spectral sensitivity of the eye is to superimpose a coloured filter. This is known as a 'colour-corrected' illuminance meter. The other method is to use correction factors, which are be provided by the manufacturer for various light sources. It is also desirable to use a light meter which is 'cosine-corrected'. Ideally all the light falling on the photocell should be measured, but light falling on the cell at an oblique angle may be reflected and not measured. To reduce these reflections a transparent hemisphere or diffusing cover is placed over the cell. Illuminance metres measuring illuminances from 0.1 to 100 000 lx, i.e. from moonlight to daylight, are available.

A luminance meter usually consists of an imaging system (some form of small telescope), a photoreceptor, and a display. The imaging system

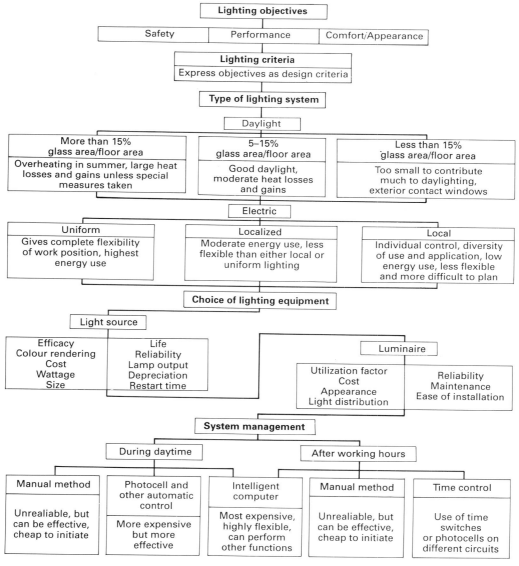

Fig 8.12 Lighting design flow chart (from the *Thorn lighting technical handbook*, courtesy of Thorn Lighting Ltd).

is adjusted so that it forms an image of the object of regard on the photocell. Like the illuminance meter, the photocell must be colour-corrected. Luminance meters that can operate over the range of 10^{-4}–10^8 cd/m² are available. They can be used for areas varying in size from a few seconds of arc up to a few degrees.

Photographic light meters can be used to estimate light levels. Once again the appropriate correction factors must be employed. For further details see Long and Woo (1980) and Smith (1982).

Summary

To summarize, this chapter has attempted to outline the major types of light sources available, their characteristics, and the various methods of lighting design. As there are so many different types of artificial light sources, and a constant flow of new developments, the choice of light source and layout can be very difficult. Figure 8.12 shows a design flow chart that gives a sequence of steps to help simplify the planning of a lighting scheme (Thorn lighting 1991).

References

BS 950 (1961). *Artificial daylight in the assessment of colour*, Part 1. BSI, London.
BS 950 (1967). *Artificial daylight in the assessment of colour*, Part 2. BSI, London.
BS 4533 (1990). *Luminaires*. BSI, London.
CIBS (1984). *Code for interior lighting*. Chartered Institute of Building Services, London.
CIBSE (1989). *Lighting guide number 2: hospitals and health care buildings*. Chartered Institute of Building Services, London.
CIBS Technical Memorandum 5. (1980). *The calculation and use of utilization factors*. Chartered Institute of Building Services, London.
CIBS Technical Memorandum 10 (1985) *Evaluation of discomfort glare—the IES Glare Index system for artificial lighting installations*. Chartered Institute of Building Services, London.
CIBS Technical Memorandum 15. (1988). *The multiple criterion design method: a design method for electric lighting installations*. Chartered Institute of Building Services, London.
EASL and LIF (1986). *Interior lighting design*, (6th edn). Electricity Association Services Ltd and Lighting Industry Federation Ltd, London.
Electricity Council (1984). *Lighting for visual inspection*. Technical Information EC 4573/5, London.
Electricity Council (1990). *Better office lighting*. Technicial Information EC 5212/1, London.
Factories Act (1961). HMSO, London.
Health and Safety at Work Act (1974). HMSO, London.
Long, W.G. and Woo, G.C.S. (1980). Measuring light levels with photographic meters. *Am. J. Optom. Physiol.* Opt., **57**, 51–5.
Pritchard, D.C. (1985). *Lighting*, (3rd edn). Longman Group Ltd, Harlow, Essex.
Smith, G. (1982). Measurement of luminance and illuminance using photographic (luminance) light meters. *Aust. J. Optom.*, **65**, 144–6.
Thorn Lighting (1991). *Thorn lighting technical handbook*, (4th edn), (ed. G. Williams). Borehamwood, Hertfordshire.

Further reading

Cayless, M.A. and Marsden, A.M. (ed.) (1983). *Lamps and lighting—a manual of lamps and lighting*, (3rd edn). Edward Arnold, London.
Lyons, S.L. (1983). *Management guide to modern industrial lighting*, (2nd edn), Butterworths, London.

Other useful publications from the Chartered Institute of Building Services, 222 Balham High Road, London SW12 9BS are:

Lighting guides for:
  Building and civil engineering sites
  Hostile and hazardous environments
  Lecture theatres
  Libraries
  Museums and art galleries
  Shipbuilding and ship-repair
  The outdoor environment

and from the Electricity Association Services Ltd, 30, Millbank, London SWIP 4RD are:

EC4465 Lighting for retailers
EC4131 Essentials of security lighting
EC3344 Outdoor lighting
EC4410 Lighting for hotels and restaurants
EC4551 Uplighters
EC4377 Lighting and low vision

9. Visual display units

Over the past few years there has been a rapid increase in the number of people using visual display units (VDUs)/terminals (VDTs) both at home and at work. The introduction of VDUs, whilst having many advantages, has unfortunately also created concern about their use and possible health hazards. This chapter outlines the data concerning health and welfare of VDU operators and the recommendations for the design of the work station and environment.

The various health risks that are associated with the use of VDUs and that may affect the eyes, are:

(1) asthenopia/eye strain;
(2) facial rash/dermatitis;
(3) epilepsy—photosensitive type;
(4) radiation.

Asthenopia

Asthenopia is a very common complaint amongst VDU operators. Some studies have estimated that up to 40 per cent of VDU operators suffer daily from asthenopic symptoms (Bergquist 1984). These symptoms may be due to a variety of factors (Chakman and Guest 1983):

(1) ocular status;
(2) personal factors;
(3) work station factors—glare, luminance, flicker, colour, contrast, alphanumeric design, and postural factors;
(4) environmental factors—room temperature, relative humidity, and air movement.

The symptoms of asthenopia may be ocular, visual, systemic, or functional. The ocular symptoms are sore, tired, tender, itchy, dry, burning, throbbing, or aching eyes. The usual visual symptoms are focusing problems, blurred or double vision, and fixation problems. The systemic symptoms are headaches and tiredness, while functional symptoms include behavioural changes.

Ocular status

VDU operators have a task that makes severe visual demands and, hence, it is not surprising that there are complaints of asthenopia. One possible reason for the asthenopia is uncorrected refractive errors. It has been estimated that about 30 per cent of the clerical workers have uncorrected or inadequately corrected visual defects (Ungar 1971). Several studies have investigated the relationship between visual defects and asthenopia in VDU operators; the results are somewhat conflicting. Gunnarson and Ostberg (1977) and Dain *et al.* (1988) found that workers with minor refractive errors, especially astigmatism, are likely to be predisposed to asthenopic symptoms. However, other studies investigating visual function and asthenopic sypmtoms do not show a consistent relationship (De Groot and Kamphuis 1983; Dainoff *et al.* 1981).

Asthenopia is also frequently caused by convergence and accommodation difficulties. Convergence insufficiency and low fusional reserves have been found to be a major cause of asthenopia amongst VDU operators (Gunnarson and Soderberg 1980). Dain *et al.* (1988) found that the horizontal near heterophoria was significantly different between asymptomatic and symptomatic VDU operators. However, no basis for a standard could be established. Inadequate accommodation may lead to asthenopia, especially amongst presbyopic operators, who may not be able to focus the required distances without an appropriate spectacle correction.

The speed of accommodation decreases with age and the layout of the VDU work station should take this into account, as the viewing distances change rapidly from script to screen to keyboard. For data-entry tasks the viewing direction is estimated to alter once very 0.8–4 s and, ideally, the keyboard, screen, and script should be positioned at the same distance from the operator, to avoid alteration of accommodation (Cakir *et al.* 1980). The use of a document holder is particularly beneficial, especially for older operators.

The accommodative search system is thought to be affected during VDU operation, as blur is a stimulus to accommodation (Fincham 1951; Phillips and Stark 1977). Dot matrix characters, which have blurred edges, may cause the accommodative system to search in an attempt to produce a clear image. Hence the focusing search with VDU displays may be higher than in non-VDU displays, e.g. script. This could lead to accommodative fatigue. However, Rupp *et al.* (1984) found no significant difference in the accommodation stability between hard copy and VDU viewing.

Transient changes in accommodation have been encountered. Osterberg (1980) found an increase in the dark focus (i.e. resting point of accommodation) indicating an increase in ciliary tonus (spasm) after VDU work. Murch (1982) also found that the accommodative system does not focus as accurately on the display as on script. The accommodation system tends to move towards the dark focus, rather than focus accurately on the plane of the VDU screen. It has therefore been suggested that the VDU screen should be positioned at a distance approaching that of the dark focus, i.e. 100–66 cm, to allow for the under-accommodation of the visual system, thus maintaining a clearer focus (Murch 1982).

After a work period of 4 h on a VDU it can take up to 15 min for the induced myopia to relax and clear distance vision to return (Holler *et al.* 1975). A recent study by Yeow and Taylor (1989) assessed both short-term and long-term changes in visual functions of VDU operators. The study revealed a small but significant myopic shift in refractive error of 0.11 D following continuous VDU usage for periods up to 4 h. This shift was seen in both presbyopic and non-presbyopic operators, and it rapidly returned to normal after the work was completed. VDU operators who were monitored for a period of 2 years did not appear to have any permanent myopic shift (Yeow 1988). Cole *et al.* (1989) are presently engaged in a 6-year study of a group of VDU operators and a control group, to determine whether VDU work does cause myopia. During the initial examination of the two groups, the VDU operators were found to be significantly more myopic than the control group (difference in mean refractive error between the groups being 0.35 D). The most likely cause for this is felt to be self-selection, i.e. myopes have some characteristic(s) that has led them to select occupations involving VDU use.

A review of the literature by Bergquist (1984) showed that, at present, there is no study that shows conclusively that a change in accommodation or oculomotor function can be attributed specifically to VDU use.

Type of work

Copy typists have a very visually demanding task. Reports indicate that they are more likely to complain of asthenopia than operators using only a VDU (Laubli *et al.* 1980). It has been found that some copy typists prefer to view the copy from the right rather than the left side because their binocular co-ordination and binocular stability are better in this viewing direction. When reading, a person tends to take a head orientation that will bias the position of the text slightly to the right of the median plane. If, therefore, text to be copied is placed in any other position, the binocular stability may well be affected (Bedwell 1978). It should also be noted that convergence is held more easily below the horizontal than above. Hence the screen and document holder should be situated below eye level.

Work breaks

The length of time spent by an operator at a VDU affects the incidence of asthenopia. For example, Gunnarsson and Soderberg (1980) found that increasing the time at the VDU from 3.5 to 6 h produced an increase from 9 to 45 per cent in the number of operators reporting symptoms. This represents a five-fold increase in the number of people with problems, which were caused by less than twice the amount of exposure.

Frequent work breaks are strongly advised to reduce the incidence of asthenopia, especially for operators who have no variation in tasks during the work period. The US National Institute of Occupational safety and Health (NOISH) recommend a 15 min work break after 2 h of continuous VDU work under moderate visual demands and/or moderate work loads or after 1 h of high visual demand, high work load, and/or repetitive work tasks (Miller 1984).

Visual standards for VDU operators

It has been suggested that companies should screen the vision of VDU operators prior to employment and at frequent intervals thereafter. This screening should be carried out to ensure that any refractive error and/or any oculomotor imbalance can be corrected to give maximum visual efficiency and comfort.

The Association of Optometrists (AOP) has suggested a specific visual standard for VDU operators for the guidance of the profession (AOP 1979).

The recommendations are as follows:

1. The ability to read N6 at a distance of 0.66 m down to 0.33 m.

2. Monocular vision or good binocular vision. Near phorias greater than 0.5 prism dioptre vertically, or 2 prism dioptres esophoria and 8 prism dioptres exophoria at working distances are contraindicated and should be corrected unless they are well compensated or deep suppression is present.

3. No central (20 degrees) field defect in the dominant eye.

4. Near point of convergence normal.

5. Clear ocular media examined by ophthalmoscopy and slit lamp.

Recommendations for minimum optometric tests have been set in other countries. In the USA, NIOSH has adapted two alternative methods, one given by the American Optometric Association and the other suggested by the National Society for the Prevention of Blindness. These recommendations, along with those of the New Zealand National Health and Medical Research Council and the Australian Optometric Association, are set out in a review by Chakman and Guest (1983). Table 9.1 summarizes some of the recommended screening procedures for VDU users (Taylor and Yeow 1990).

Most of the recommendations do not include a measurement of the fusional reserves or fixation disparity. As asthenopia or blurred vision is often due to the inability to compensate for a heterophoria due to poor fusion, it would be of significant value to measure the fusional reserves and the fixation disparity. The latter can indicate the stress in the binocular system and it has been reported to show an exo-shift after a day of close work (Yekta *et al.* 1987). Whilst the various standards for VDU operators require the heterophoria to be within certain logical limits, they have not been based on clinical studies. Another point to note is that some of the recommendations do not include ophthalmoscopy, which is necessary for the early detection of ocular pathology.

Ideally, the vision screening should be carried out by a qualified person and should include ophthalmoscopy and retinoscopy either as part of a full examination or as a modified clinical technique. Although it is more expensive to employ a professional person, the number of false referrals will be reduced and the reliability of the results assured. Vision re-checks should be carried out at regular intervals; a two-yearly period has been suggested by the Australian Optometric Association.

Table 9.1 Recommended screening procedures for VDU operators (reproduced by courtesy of Taylor and Yeow and *The Optician* 1990)

	AOP	Australian Optometric Association	Australian National Health and Medical Research Council	UK VDU eye test Advisory Group	National Society for Prevention of Blindness	American Optometric Association
External examination of the eye	*	*				*
Ophthalmoscopy	*	*				*
Amplitude of accommodation	*	*		*		*
Suppression	*			*		
Muscle balance (distance)	*	*		*	*	*
Muscle balance (1 m)	*			*	*	*
Muscle balance (near)	*		*		*	*
Convergence	*	*		*		*
Refraction—distance	*		*	*	*	*
Refraction—intermediate	*			*		*
Refraction—near	*		*	*	*	*
Colour vision		*	*		*	*
Visual fields		*				*
Tonometry		*				*
Retinoscopy		*				*
Unaided acuity				*		
Stereopsis		*			*	*
Keratometry						*

If an instrument screener is to be used then care should be taken to select one which includes an intermediate testing distance. For a summary of the available vision screeners, see Chapter 2. An alternative method of vision screening is to use a computerized test programme. Software packages are presently being designed that can be used by the operators at their own work stations. The results of the vision screening are automatically evaluated and a printout is provided. One advantage of this type of screening is that tests are carried out under the actual work conditions.

Spectacle prescriptions

An emmetropic pre-presbyope should not have any problem in focusing the range of distances required for VDU work. The VDU screen may be situated at a distance of 50–70 cm whilst the keyboard and often the script is usually at a closer distance of approximately 33–40 cm. Figure 9.1(a) shows the typical focusing abilities of various age groups. Whereas a 30-year-old can focus at all the necessary distances without any problem, an operator in their mid-forties will be able to read the VDU screen easily but may have difficulty reading scripts/if they are positioned at a closer distance. A 50-year-old operator may have difficulty in focusing on both the VDU screen and the scripts without a spectacle prescription.

Problems occur for the presbyopic operator in that a conventional near correction for 40 cm is often too restrictive. Figure 9.1(b) shows the range of clear vision of older operators wearing spectacle prescription for reading only. For a 60-year-old, the keyboard and script will be in focus but the VDU screen will be blurred. To enable the older operator to read both the screen and the script, spectacles specially for use with a VDU may have to be prescribed.

Grundy and Rosenthal (1982) have found that the straight line bifocals (i.e. so-called executive (E) or D segments) are superior to round or crescent-top bifocals, (Fig. 9.2). They provide a greater area of useful vision and, therefore, minimize head and eye movements. Also, there is a reduction of 'jump'—displacement of objects—which occurs when viewing is changed from one section of the lens to the other. However, operators up to the age of 50 years may find conventional bifocals suitable, although the bifocal segment height may need to be increased to correspond to the position of the VDU screen. It is suggested that the ideal situation for viewing the VDU screen is with the eyes depressed at an angle of 15–20 degrees from the horizontal. Older operators (over 50 years of age) may require an intermediate and near prescription. This can be provided by bifocals in which the upper part of the lens provides an intermediate prescription to focus the screen and the lower segment contains a near prescription to focus the script if it is positioned nearer than the screen. However, if the screen and script are placed at the same distance then operators often cope well with an intermediate single vision prescription. Trifocal lenses can be used if clear distance vision is required. Particularly useful are trifocals with distance and intermediate Executive lenses with a D segment for the near prescription, e.g. SE 825, SE 1128.

The use of progressive lenses is controversial. Some authors consider them to be less suitable than bifocals, especially when a script to be copied is placed at the side of the VDU. They have a smaller reading area and can produce unwanted peripheral distortions. They also require considerable head movement for VDU work. When viewing the screen the operator usually looks through the intermediate zone of the lens, which is relatively narrow and set low, requiring the head to be tilted back. Whilst the width of the zone may be adequate for most visual needs of daily life it is not entirely satisfactory for VDU work. Therefore some reject progresssive lenses because of the forced head posture, resultant neck cramp, and limitations of the intermediate and near portions' size

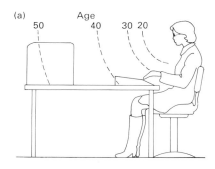

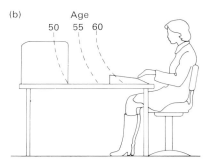

Fig. 9.1 (a) The focusing ability varying with age. The dotted lines indicate the closest point at which near tasks can be viewed for prolonged periods of time without wearing spectacles prescribed for near. (b) The resticted range of clear vision of older operators wearing spectacle prescribed only for reading. Dotted lines indicate point beyond which vision will be blurred (reproduced by kind permission of Grundy et al. and The Association of Optometrists (1991).

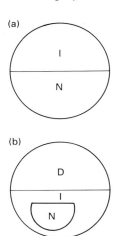

Fig. 9.2 Examples of some of the lens forms available for presbyopic VDU operators. (a) Executive bifocal; (b) trifocal. D, distance prescription; I, intermediate prescription; and N, near prescription.

upon vision. However, more recent progressive lenses have been designed specifically for VDU operators, e.g. Technica (UKO) and Datacomfort (Essilor). These have larger intermediate areas which are set slightly higher than conventional progressive lenses and allows the centre of the intermediate vision to be in the middle of the area situated between 10 and 20 degrees below the horizontal. Horgen *et al.* (1989) studied the effects of bifocals and progressive lenses upon the muscle load in the neck/shoulder region and on working posture. They confirmed that single vision lenses create less trapesium load than multifocals. However, if the operator requires multifocals then the work station must be ergonomically designed. The results also suggested that lowering the near segments of the multifocals 2 mm below the manufacturer's recommendation reduced the trapezium load. This finding conflicts with common clinical opinion, which is that the near segments should be fitted higher than normal for VDU operators.

Hamard *et al.* (1987) studied emmetropic presbyopic VDU operators, who were given half-eye spectacles fitted with Varilux 2 lenses positioned so that the intermediate progression started at the upper edge of the frame. These were found to be particularly successful allowing good horizontal and vertical scanning. Another study (Good and Daum 1985) also investigated the use of half-eye spectacles fitted with progressive lenses. They recommended that emmetropes can be fitted with progressive lenses incorporating a +0.75 D addition to the distance power and with the near power appropriately reduced; this increases the intermediate and near focusing portions of the lens. After an initial adaptation period most wearers reacted favourably to these lenses. A half-eye frame with a large vertical dimension is advised to allow full use of the near addition.

Contact lenses have an advantage over spectacles in that they give rise to fewer reflections and distortions. However, problems may occur due to the fact that concentration on the VDU, or any task for that matter, often results in a reduced blink rate, which will cause symptoms resembling those of a 'dry eye'. The tear film can also be affected by high temperatures and low humidity, which may result in similar symptoms.

Several companies have introduced VDU spectacles with tinted lenses. These were designed to reduce asthenopia by reducing glare from overhead light sources, windows, or the VDU screen; they also claim to improve the contrast of the characters on the screen. For example, American Optical (AO) produced three tints that can be made up in prescription form if required. These decrease internal lens reflections by > 60 per cent and absorb the majority of ambient UV light. Magenta-tinted lenses have been designed for viewing VDUs with green-emitting phosphor, grey for black and white, and blue for amber displays.

The Rodenstock company has also designed a lens to reduce the glare associated with VDU work. The upper part of the lens is tinted green to cut out direct or reflected glare. The green tint has 60 per cent absorption.

Obstfeld and Thomson (1985) reviewed some of the tinted lenses introduced to reduce glare. They concluded that because VDUs do not emit much radiation in the UV or IR parts of the spectrum, tinted lenses that

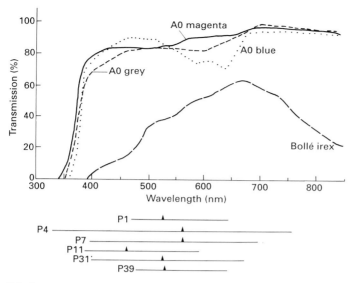

Fig. 9.3 Spectral transmission curves of some VDU lenses. Phophor colours: P1, P7, and P39, yellowish green; P4, white; P11, blue; and P31, green (reproduced by kind permission of Obstfeld and Thomson and *Optometry Today* 1985).

absorb these wavelengths will not be of much use. To reduce glare and hence enhance contrast, the spectral transmissions of the tinted lenses should be matched to the spectral emissions of the VDU screen phospors. Figure 9.3 shows that the AO and Bolle Irex 90+ filters do not have transmission curves that match the commonly employed screen phosphors. The most likely effect of these filters is to diminish the contrast of the display.

Mousa (1986) studied the effects of tinted lenses (pink and UV-absorbing) on the spectral distribution from fluorescent lights, which are found in most office areas. Results indicated that both lenses will reduce the discomfort caused by stray light, but by different methods. The pink lenses will reduce the overall illumination, which is suggested to be useful as most offices are over-illuminated for VDU operation, whilst the UV-absorbing lenses eliminate UV, which is scattered by the cornea and lens.

To conclude, it would be best to try to control/eliminate the glare sources wherever possible, before prescribing tinted VDU spectacles.

Personal factors

Factors such as general fatigue, ill health, the use of certain drugs, and a tendency to migraine and photophobia are some of the physiological factors that may contribute to symptoms of eye strain. Psychological factors, such as nervous or anxious personality, level of stress, motivation, and interest in the work may also be associated with eye strain. Although these personal factors may increase the risk of asthenopic symptoms arising, the physical factors of the environment and task are generally the main cause.

Trainee VDU operators may well complain of asthenopia because they must maintain high level of concentration and because unfamiliar demands are made upon the visual system. Once the operator has become acquainted with the VDU and its operation the symptoms will generally decrease, provided that the design, environment, etc., of the VDU is correct.

It has been suggested that older VDU operators will complain more of asthenopia. The results of various studies are conflicting, some finding that the younger operators complain more of asthenopia (Starr *et al*. 1982; Sauter 1984) whilst others find the reverse or no difference (Rey and Meyer 1980; Levy and Ramberg 1987; Ong and Phoon 1987). There are significantly more complaints regarding health and asthenopic symptoms from women operators (Murray *et al*. 1981; Knave *et al*. 1985).

Several studies have investigated stress among VDU operators. Stress commonly arises when the person's perception of their own abilities are not matched by the job's demands. This is a frequent complaint reported by VDU operators, who perform repetitive, monotonous tasks. Data entry seems to be particularly responsible for many adverse health effects (Salvendy 1982; Knave and Wideback 1987; Levy and Ramberg 1987).

To minimize stress for the VDU operators, the task should therefore be designed to avoid or reduce repetitive elements by introducing variability in the workload, instead of long periods of concentrated work. Ideally, the change from conventional office handling routines to VDU-based systems should provide an opportunity to experience job satisfaction by removing the repetitive, simple tasks.

Work Station Design

Factors to be considered in work station design are: lighting, glare, flicker, colour contrast, alpha–numeric design; and ergonomics.

Lighting

The correct level of illumination is essential for a comfortable and efficient visual performance. Several investigators have suggested that illumination and its effects on the VDU are a possible cause of the high rate of asthenopic symptoms amongst the operators (Hultgren and Knave 1974; Gunnarsson and Ostberg 1977; Cakir *et al*. 1980). A high level of illumination will improve the legibility of the script when there are dark characters on a light background, but the reverse occurs for a display with light characters on a dark screen. Therefore, an optimum level of illumination is required to ensure that the legibility of the script and the screen characters are least impaired. CIBSE (1989), Lighting guide for visual display terminals, recommends a background illuminance level of 300–500 lx. The lower end of the range should be used when the task is mainly screen-based, e.g. data retrieval, and the upper end of the range should be used when the task is mainly documentation-based, e.g. data entry. Different illumination levels were assessed subjectively by VDU operators and the majority found their task easiest at levels of around 300 lx (Varrall 1983). Older VDU operators will require a higher level of illumination, which can be provided by local lighting but must be shielded from other operators, or it will act as a glare source. In general, ambient

Table 9.2 Categories of downlighter luminaires for VDUs (from CIBSE 1989)

Category	VDU use	Luminance limitation angle	Other uses
1	Intense	55 degrees	High density area of VDUs. Older types of VDUs. Highly specular surfaces
2	General	65 degrees	Positive contrast displays
3	Minimal	75 degrees	Low density area of VDUs. Positive contrast displays

The angles do not refer to cut off angles but a sharp run back on the polar curve in all vertical planes. Above these angles the average luminance does not exceed 200 cd/m^2.

lighting should provide about two—thirds of the required illuminance and local lighting of the work station should provide the rest.

The lighting needs to be designed to avoid direct and reflected glare and this can be achieved by direct lighting from low-luminance downward-pointing luminaires, by direct lighting from uplighters, or by a combination of the two systems.

The CIBSE (1989) guide defines three categories of luminaires for downlighters depending on the degree of VDU use: (i) intense VDU use; (ii) general VDU use; and (iii) minimal VDU use. It is hoped that manufacturers will state the category that their luminaires fall into. Table 9.2 details the categories of downlighters. The recommended room reflectances, with/without daylight, are: (i) floor, 0.3/0.2; (ii) work surface, 0.4/0.3; (iii) walls, 0.5/0.5; and (iv) ceiling, 0.7/0.7.

When using uplighters, the ceiling is used as a large area of low luminance. This overcomes any problems of glare; any reflections from the VDU screen will be of low luminance. Uplighters can be free floor-standing, furniture-mounted, wall-mounted, or suspended and, ideally, they should be used where the ceiling height is at least 2.5 m. According to CIBS (1989) the room reflectances, especially that of the ceiling, should be 0.8. The average luminance of the ceiling, or other major reflecting surfaces, should be less than 500 cd/m^2 and should not be greater than 15 000 cd/m^2 at any point. Various light sources are suitable for uplighters. The metal halide lamps and high pressure sodium lamps can be used in all forms of uplighters; tubular and compact fluorescent lamps are large and are therefore used in the furniture-mounted or suspended forms.

Glare

Glare, as already mentioned, is one of main complaints made by VDU operators and is caused by bright sources of light falling within the operator's field of vision. There are two types of glare: (i) disability glare; and (ii) discomfort glare (see p. 152). The former impairs the ability to see detail without necessarily causing visual discomfort and the latter causes visual discomfort without impairing the ability to see detail. To avoid discomfort glare a glare index of 19 is recommended for general office work (CIBS 1984). Values of this order or less can be achieved if the area is lit according to the recommendations in CIBSE (1989).

Glare may arise from direct light or, indirectly, from reflections. Direct glare is most frequently caused by the light from a window or an artificial light source that is too large or too bright. Other causes of glare are reflections from shiny, even surfaces such as gloss-painted walls, linoleum covered floor, polished wooden furniture, etc. Light may be reflected from the VDU itself from the screen or the keyboard. Reflectances from the surface of the VDU screen can be very annoying. Screens are often slightly convex and act as a mirror, reflecting whatever is in front of the screen, e.g. the operator or light sources. The concave keys can also reflect light into the operators eyes.

There are several methods of reducing or eliminating glare sources (Birnbaum 1978; CIBSE 1989; Grundy *et al.* 1991):

1. Adjust the position of the VDU screen so that the operator cannot see any reflections from the screen or other polished surfaces.
2. Change the position of troublesome light sources where possible.
3. Fit light sources with the appropriate diffusers.
4. Fluorescent light fittings, if used, should be positioned with their length parallel to the side of the VDU.
5. The screen should be non-reflective and designed so that it can be tilted or rotated.
6. The keyboard should have a matt surround and the keys should have low reflectance surfaces.
7. Matt scripts should be used, preferably in pastel colours.
8. Use a light-coloured desk top in preference to a dark one.
9. The VDU has contrast and brightness controls so that the legibility of the characters on the screen can be altered. The ratio of luminances between the work station and the immediate surrounding should be within a range of 1 to 10 (CIBSE 1989).
10. Windows should be fitted with blinds, e.g. vertical louvred blinds.

Several methods have been used to try and eliminate the screen reflections (Cakir *et al.* 1980): (i) filter panels; (ii) polarization filters; (iii) micromesh filters; (iv) etching the glass screen; (v) anti-reflection coats—vapour-deposited 0.25 wavelength thin film; and (vi) tube shields.

Each type of filter has advantages and disadvantages, which may vary depending upon the environment. Unfortunately, many of the techniques, whilst decreasing the amount of reflected light, also reduce the character brightness and resolution.

Cakir *et al.* (1980) have suggested that, in a normal office environment, filters can be ranked in decreasing order of effectiveness: (i) Anti-reflection coating; (ii) etching; (iii) polarization with additional anti-reflection layer; (iv) micromesh filters; and (v) polarization filter. The best method of providing an anti-reflection coating without losing the clarity of the characters is by the vacuum deposition of a thin film layer with a thickness of 0.25 the wavelength of light. This technique is effective but expensive, as the coating is applied to a glass panel, which is then bonded to the screen surface. It is also very sensitive to dust and dirt, and shows up finger prints. Therefore, if the filter surface is not cleaned regularly the characters will appear to be smeared.

Flicker

A flickering image on a screen will diminish the legibility and cause fatigue and asthenopia, depending upon the length of time that the screen is viewed. The flicker on the VDU screen is dependent upon design characteristics of the display and personal factors. The design characteristics to be taken into account include the phosphor type, refresh rate, character size and colour, area of screen illuminated, and viewing angle. The personal factors include the critical fusion frequency (CFF) and tolerance to a flickering display. The CFF is the lowest frequency at which a flickering stimulus is perceived as continuous. It varies between individuals and is affected by such factors as pupil size, age, and general health.

The characters on a VDU screen are generated by electrons. The screen is coated with phosphor which, when bombarded with electrons, produces a spot of light. The intensity and position of the spot can be controlled so that characters can be formed. The rate at which the phosphorescent image decays (0.001–1 s) and the rate at which it is refreshed by the electronic pulse is very important. If the pulse refresh rate is slow (30–40 Hz) and the decay rate is fast due to a short duration phoshor, the normal saccadic and the minor oscillatory eye movements will interact with the intermittent image formation, causing different parts of the retina to be stimulated. This will result in the display appearing to 'jump' along the line in the case of saccadic eye movements and to 'dance' in the case of eye tremors (Birnbaum 1978). Long persistence phosphors decrease the 'jump' and 'dance' of the display but have a short life and produce 'smearing' of the characters. This smearing is caused by the persistent after–image when the character is changed.

The use of dark characters on a light background (positive contrast or polarity) ensures good legibility, as reflections are less obvious and edges of the characters appear sharper. However, positive contrast tends to enhance the flicker effect. It has therefore been suggested that negative contrast displays should be used (Miller 1984). These have another advantage in that the legibility is superior for people with low vision (CIBSE 1989).

Research has suggested that refresh rates of up to 100 Hz may be needed to avoid flicker of some high luminance displays (Bauer *et al.* 1983).

There are several methods available for calculating the refresh rate for a screen to appear flicker-free which take into account such factors as the type of phosphor, luminance, and size of the screen (ISO 9241, BS 7179). Using a simplified method, the International Standards Organization (ISO 9241) suggest that a 72 Hz display will appear flicker-free. This standard is being finalized and will be adopted as the European standard on completion.

Colour contrast

Colour contrast is not essential in determining the legibility of a display; it is the overall contrast that is more important. The colour of the phosphors

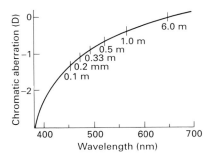

Fig. 9.4 Axial chromatic aberrations of the eye (reproduced by kind permission of Sivak JC, Woo GC, Colour of visual display terminals and the eye. Green VDTs provide optimal stimulus to accommodation. Am. J. Optom. Physiol. Opt. 60(7):640–641. (c) The American Academy of Optometry, 1983).

used for VDUs varies. Green phosphors are usually used for monochromatic displays as they are most readily available. From surveys it appears that white, yellow, or green on a neutral background are the preferred combinations, with green being favoured most of all. The reason for the preference for green phosphor is the relationship between accommodation and chromatic aberration. It has been shown that the wavelength in focus on the retina varies with the state of accommodation. When the eye is unaccommodated, and fixating a distant target, a wavelength of about 650 nm is in focus (Millodot and Sivak 1973). However, when the eye accommodates for targets at closer distances, the wavelength in focus gradually shifts towards the short wavelengths. At a distance of 0.5 m the wavelength in focus is about 520 nm, i.e. green phosphors P1, P31, and P39 (max 525–520 nm) would be most suitable (Fig. 9.4). Blue phosphors, e.g. P11 (max 460 nm) would induce a small amount of myopia if the operator accommodates by the amount normally appropriate for 0.5 m (Sivak and Woo 1983).

Scrolling

It is possible to generate scrolling on a VDU screen so that the text moves rapidly up the screen. It has been suggested that increased rates of scrolling lead to poor performance and increased stress (Barfield 1984).

Alpha–numeric displays

The characters on the displays should be:

1. Visible. Characters should be readily detectable from the background.
2. Legible. It should be easy to identify each character.
3. Readable. Spacing of characters, etc. should permit easy reading. Careful consideration has to be given to the design of the various features of the characters and their arrangement.

The following factors should be considered regarding the legibility of characters:

CHARACTER FORMAT

Each character is composed of a matrix of circular dots. The greater the number of dots the better the quality of the character. Problems arise with a 5×7 (width to height) matrix as it is difficult to distinguish between certain numerals and letters, such as U and V, S and 5, and therefore, more operator errors are likely. For this reason the 7×9 matrix is most commonly used. The size of the dots is also important: if they are too small the character has a broken appearance and, if too large, it is difficult to resolve. A technique for enhancing the characters and giving them a more rounded appearance is known as 'half-shift' (Fig. 9.5) whereby some of the dots are moved in the horizontal plane, by half a dot separation, to the left or right (Reading 1978).

BS 7179 (1990) makes the following recommendations regarding the character format:

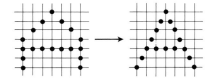

Fig. 9.5 Character formation by dot matrices. The appearance can be enhanced by displacing some of the dots horizontally by a half dot separation.

1. A 7×9 matrix should be the minimum used for tasks requiring continuous reading for context or in tasks such as proof reading, where legibility of each character is important.

2. A 5×7 matix should be the minimum used for numeric and upper case only presentations.

3. A 4×5 matrix should be used for superscripts and for numerators and denominators of fractions that are to be displayed in a single character position.

CHARACTER HEIGHT

It is suggested that the minimum mean character height shall be 16 min of arc; the preferred height for most tasks being between 20–22 min of arc (BS 7179 1990).

HEIGHT TO WIDTH RATIO

The relationship between the height and width of a character is usually described as the height to width ratio. BS 7179 (1990) suggests a ratio of between 1.05 and 1.1 for proportionally spaced characters and between 1.07 and 1.09 for character sets not proportionally spaced.

STROKE WIDTH TO HEIGHT RATIO

The stroke width is the width of the line forming the letter or symbol. It is usually expressed as the ratio of the thickness of the stroke to the height of the character. BS 7179 (1990) recommends a stroke width of between one-sixth and one-twelfth of the character height. It also suggests that wider strokes are preferred for dark characters on a white background (positive polarity). White characters on black (negative polarity) can have a thinner stroke width as the white appears to spread to the adjacent black; the converse is not true.

The characters and lines should be well spaced for easy reading. The inter-character spacing must be such that an adequate number of characters can be viewed with a single fixation of the eye. BS 7179 (1990) suggests that:

1. The between-character spacing shall be a minimum of one stroke width or one pixel, whichever is greater (for fonts without serifs).

2. The between-word spacing shall be a minimum of one character.

3. The between-line spacing shall be a minimum of one stroke width or pixel, whichever is greater.

Most VDUs have a line width of 80 characters, whereas a script has 60 characters per line. As the display should not cause unnecessary fatigue, overcrowding and cramming of letters within lines should be avoided. If the task involves continuous text, upper and lower case letters should be used (Reading 1978).

DISPLAY LUMINANCE AND CONTRAST

BS 7179 (1990) suggests that the display shall be capable of a luminance of at least 35 cd/m^2 and that the minimum luminance contrast of character details relevant for legibility shall be at least 3 : 1.

Ergonomics

To ensure that the design of the work station is operational, the VDU operator should:

(1) have easy access and regress;

(2) be able to reach and operate all controls with ease;

(3) be able to see and reach all the displays;

(4) be able to work comfortably.

The very common complaints of back- and neck-ache may be due to incorrect work station design, perhaps due to chair position or the height/angle of the VDU being fixed without any method of adjustment/alteration.

The relationship between poor posture and eyestrain/asthenopia is controversial. Some argue that poor posture will cause fatigue of the neck and back, and hence lead to ocular fatigue/asthenopia. Others argue that visual difficulties lead to poor posture. Bergquist (1984) reviewed the literature on this subject and concluded that musculoskeletal problems are not specific to VDU operators, and are found in people doing other types of office work. However, the site of discomfort appears to be different. VDU operators appear to suffer more from discomfort in the neck, shoulders, and upper arms, whilst non-VDU-operators complain more of pain in the extremities. The occurrence of musculoskeletal pain is found more frequently in women, in people engaged in data entry, and after long periods of work.

Screen

According to the Health and Safety Executive (HSE) (1983) the VDU screen should positioned at a distance of 35–60 cm from the operator (70 cm maximum). Ideally, the eyes should be depressed at an angle of 15–20 degrees. The screen should be at right angles to the line of sight and it should be possible to rotate the screen laterally so that the operator is not disturbed by their own reflection. BS 7179 (1990) suggests that displays that are lower than the seated eye height and within 60 degrees of the horizontal line of sight are acceptable.

Keyboard

The keyboard height should be such that the operator's arms form angles of about 90 degrees at the elbow and allow the wrists to be slightly flexed (BS 7179 1990). Ideally, the keyboard should be detachable, to allow the operator to find the best working position, e.g. it should not be placed too far from the desk edge as this results in a cutting action by that edge on the wrists and forearms. For tasks in which largely numeric data are being entered, an auxillary numeric key set should be considered. The keyboard should have a slight slope and it should be as thin as possible. The keyboard should also have a matt surround and keys should have low reflectance surfaces (HSE 1983; Miller 1984).

Posture

The chair should have an adjustable seat height, adjustable back rest height and an adjustable tension on the back rest. The seat height should be such that the operator's legs form an angle equal to or greater than 90 degrees at the knee, with feet on the floor. This is generally achieved with the seat height being between 34 and 52 cm (HSE 1983). There should also be an adequate knee clearance between the seat and the table.

WORK TABLES AND DESKS

There should be sufficient space for documents, books, and other ancillary equipment to be arranged as required. BS 7179 (1990) suggests that the work surface should be a minimum of 120 cm long and 60 cm wide, preferably 160 cm long and 80 cm wide. The work surfaces should also have a matt finish to prevent troublesome reflectances or glare. Document holders should be provided because they will prevent bending of the neck by the operator to read documents placed flat on the desk. The holders should be adjustable and can be placed next to the VDU screen at a similar angle, distance, and height to give visual comfort.

The typical dimensions and surface reflectances of a work station according to BS 7179 (1990) Part5 are summarized in Figure 9.6.

Environmental conditions

Office decor needs to be visually restful and glare-free. High reflectance walls, ceiling, or floor surfaces may lead to glare, but low reflectance surfaces may create gloom. Therefore, large surface areas should be decorated in soft pastels or warm grey, i.e. have medium reflectance and low contrast. During extended periods of writing and reading, etc., unconscious involuntary relief for the eyes occurs by looking away from the task at distant objects. Paintings and foliage may be useful to provide visual relief.

Noisy equipment, such as printers, should be positioned away from the operator, or soundproofed. A noisy terminal should be serviced by the supplier.

VDUs and light sources inevitably produce heat which, in warm weather or in confined spaces, can become a real problem if the ventilation system is not able to cope. Many VDU operators complain of sore, dry eyes. This is generally due to a reduced blink rate, which occurs with intense concentration, and to the lack of humidity, which is quite prevalent in many offices, especially those with air conditioning. This is particularly problematical for contact lens wearers. Therefore, adequate ventilation

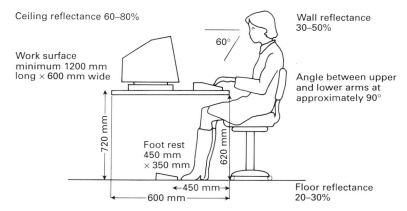

Fig. 9.6 Typical dimension and surface reflectances of a VDU work station according to BS 7179 (1990).

and reasonable humidity should be maintained to avoid such problems as drowsiness and dryness of the eyes.

BS 7179 (1990) Part 6 provides a code of practice for the design of VDU work environments and includes recommendations for lighting, surface reflectances, noise levels, and thermal conditions. HSE (1983) and CIBSE (1989) also detail environmental conditions.

Facial rash/dermatitis

There are several reports concerning facial rashes amongst VDU operators (Rycroft and Calnan 1980; Tjonn 1980). The complaints varied from itching of the skin to reddening with occasional minor desquamation and small papules. It usually occurs after a couple of hours at work and disappears a few hours after leaving work.

All VDUs generate a positively charged electrostatic field, which extends 2–3 m in front of the VDU. This field is generated by the interaction of the electron beam with the VDU screen and attracts particles of smoke, pollen, and dust, etc. These particles are then drawn to the nearest negative charge, or ground, which may be the face or hands of the operator. Negatively charged particles will also be drawn to the screen, forming the commonly seen 'dusty' layer.

Various experiments have been carried out to prevent skin reactions amongst known cases. One method tried was to place a glass sheet between the operator and the screen. The results have been conflicting. One case reported the method to be successful whilst another found it of no use in preventing the facial rash. The most successful method appears to be the elimination of build-up of static electricity by replacing normal floor carpets with anti-static carpets and by the grounding of the display terminals (Cakir *et al.* 1980; HSE 1983). It is believed that the contact dermatitis is caused by irritating submicron dust particles precipitating on the skin of the VDU operator because they are accumulating static electricity. Manufacturers should try to design the unit so that the outside screen potential is as near to 0V as possible. Periodic cleaning of the VDU screen with anti-static solution will control the dust accumulation and maintaining a constant relative humidity of 50–70 per cent should also help (Canadian Occupational Environment Branch of the Ministry of Labour 1983).

Epilepsy

There has been concern in the past about people who suffer from epilepsy operating VDUs. In fact, VDU work does not cause epilepsy and a person who suffers from this disorder should not be prevented from being a VDU operator (HSE 1983). However, some people suffer from a relatively rare form of epilepsy, known as photosensitive epilepsy. In these people a seizure may be triggered after stimulation by a flickering light source or after viewing striped patterns. The incidence of epilepsy in the population is estimated to be about 2 per cent, of whom approximately 4 per cent suffer from photosensitive epilepsy (Wilkins 1978). Most of the people who are likely to suffer from an attack will have done so before the age of 20 years and it will probably occur whilst watching television.

The possibility of a striped pattern triggering a seizure depends on various stimulus parameters, such as: (i) area of retina stimulated; (ii) the number of cycles of the pattern per degree (typically 1–4 cycles per degree); (iii) luminance; and (iv) pattern stability (frequencies of 20 Hz should be avoided). Wilkins (1978) suggested that the epileptogenic factors of a television or VDU can be reduced by:

1. Using a small screen to reduce the area of retina stimulated.
2. Using white alphanumerics on a black background.
3. Limiting the amount of text on the screen.
4. Avoiding scrolling of the text.
5. Reducing the luminance of the display, either by the operator wearing tinted spectacles or by covering the screen with tinted perspex.

Despite this information it is still difficult to give an accurate assessment of the risk of a photosensitive epileptic suffering a seizure when operating a VDU. Thus it would be wise for a known photosensitive epileptic to seek medical advice before using VDUs. In the UK, such advice can be given by the Employment Medical Advisory Service.

Radiation

There has been a great deal of concern about dangerous radiation emissions from VDUs. According to Marriott and Stuchly (1986) radiation may be given off by:

(1) the screen (visible, UV, and IR, depending on the phosphor);
(2) the cathode tube or electronic damper circuit (X-rays);
(3) the electronic components or circuit (microwave, UV, radio-frequency).

A number of surveys have been carried out to determine the levels of electromagnetic radiation emmitted by the VDU (Weiss and Peterson 1979; Cox 1980; Terrana *et al.* 1980; Elliot *et al.* 1986). These surveys concluded that the measured values of electromagnetic radiation were at levels substantially below existing limits. The national and international limits for continuous exposure were not exceeded and, hence, the radiation emitted from VDUs is not considered to be a health hazard. For reviews of these studies see Cox (1983) and Rosner and Belkin (1989).

Regulations regarding the use of visual display units

The EC has issued legislation regarding the minimum safety and health requirements for work with display screen equipment (EC Directive 1990). Each member state can decide how the directive is implemented and in the UK the Health and Safety (Display Screen Equipment) Regulations 1992 have been issued. A booklet, *Display screen equipment work— guidance on regulations*, has been published by the Health and Safety

Executive. This is exceedingly useful as it states the regulations and then gives further information and advice in relation to the specific requirements.

It should be noted that there are other new directives which apply to all places and types of work which need to be taken into account, whether or not VDUs are being used: The Management of Health and Safety at Work Regulations, Provision and Use of Work Equipment Regulations, and Workplace (Health Safety and Welfare) Regulations.

The Health and Safety (DSE) Regulations gives definitions of 'display screen equipment', 'work station' and 'user' which determine the application of the regulations. A 'user' is stated as being an employee who habitually uses display screen equipment (DSE) as a significant part of their normal work. The term 'operator' is used for self-employed workers. Display screen equipment covered by the regulations include not only the conventional VDU but also other displays such as the microfiche and liquid crystal. But the regulations do not apply if the main use is for television or film display. There are exemptions to the regulations such as DSE intended mainly for public use and those systems used in transport, cash registers and calculator displays.

The protection applies to users whether they work at their own or other employer's work stations or at a work station at home. Employers have to decide which of their employees are 'users' and the guidelines and examples given will be of considerable help. Factors that should be taken into account are the dependence on the DSE, training required, time spent at DSE, intensity of use, and consequences of any errors. Examples of jobs are given which categorize the workers as definite users and not users according to these factors.

Analysis of the work stations must be carried out by the employer to assess the risk to the health and safety of the user. The possible risks are listed in the Appendix and the main ones are considered to be muscoskeletal problems, visual fatigue and mental stress. Any potential risks that are identified have to be dealt with straight away; the 4 year period allowed from 31 December 1992 to bring existing work stations up to the requirements does not apply in this case. Records of work station assessments and any alterations/modifications that are required should be kept.

The regulations also detail employers duties in the provision of health and safety training and information to users of work stations. The employer must also organize the daily work routine so that users are not continually operating DSE but have periodic breaks.

The minimum requirements for the work station are stated in the schedule of the regulations. It covers requirements for the DSE and the work environment including details regarding the display screen, keyboard, the work surface, chair, lighting, glare, heating, humidity, and noise. For example, the screen image must be stable and flicker-free and reflections and glare should be avoided. In the guidance it states that employers may find standards such as BS 7179 (1990) and other international standards useful. However, there is no requirement in the Display Screen Equipment Regulations for BS 7179 (1990) to be complied with. But if work stations do comply with BS 7179 then they will meet or exceed the minimum requirements set out in the schedule to the regulations. BS

7179 will be withdrawn once the European standards organization issues its standard (EN 29241).

Of particular importance for optometrists is Regulation 5. It states that the employer must provide an appropriate eye and eyesight test to employees who are existing users or to those who are to become users. Further eye and eyesight tests should be provided at regular intervals or if the user experiences visual problems which may be due to DSE work. The guidelines state that an 'eye and eyesight test' is a 'sight test' as defined by the Opticians Act. An employer may offer vision screening tests; however, if the employee requests a sight test this must be provided. There is no obligation for an employee to participate in any form of vision testing, it is entirely his/her choice.

The regulations also state that an employer must provide special protective appliances for DSE work where a sight test has shown the need and normal appliances cannot be used. For example, an intermediate prescription may be required for the screen to be seen clearly. It is estimated that only approximately 10% of the employees will require correction specifically for DSE use. The guidelines state that anti-glare screens and so called VDU spectacles are not considered to be special corrective appliances.

The British College of Optometrists (BCO) and the Association of Optometrists have each issued a statement of good practice for work with DSE. The guidelines refer to the BCO statement regarding the optometrists actions upon completion of the sight test. A report should be given to the employer with a copy to the employee stating whether or not a corrective appliance is required specifically for DSE work and when a retest is advised. The prescription for the corrective appliance can only be included in the report to the employer with the employees' permission. Also the BCO states that clinical information should only be provided to an employer if it is relevant to the employees' DSE work and only with the employees' permission. The employer is responsible for the expenses incurred in the provision of eye and eyesight tests and the provision of special corrective appliances if required. The guidelines state that the employer is liable for the costs of a basic appliance. If the user wishes a more costly appliance then the employer may contribute a portion of the total cost equivalent to that of the cost of the basic appliance.

Summary

The use of VDUs can be of great benefit in the work situation, but the visual capabilities of the operator must be assessed and the work station must be arranged in an appropriate manner to prevent the frequent complaints of asthenopia. Figure 9.7 gives a summary of some of the causes of asthenopia. If a VDU operator complains of asthenopia and requests an eye examination then the following information will prove useful in ascertaining the cause (Grundy *et al.* 1991):

(1) date of last eye exaination;

(2) when was VDU work commenced;

(3) how many hours per day of VDU use;

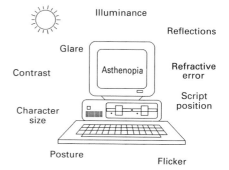

Fig. 9.7 Summary of some of the causes of asthenopia.

(4) whether work breaks are provided, and their duration;

(5) character size and form (letters, numbers) on screen and documents;

(6) colour of characters and screen;

(7) distance of screen, keyboard, and documents;

(8) position of VDU screen (above or below eye level);

(9) position of document relative to the screen;

(10) type and colour of background behind screen;

(11) reflections or glare sources in view;

(12) is the chair adjustable.

Acknowledgement

Extracts from BS 7179 (1990) are reproduced with the permission of BSI. Complete copies of the standard can be obtained from BSI Sales, Linford Wood, Milton Keynes MK14 6LE, UK.

References

AOP (1979). Recommended AOP procedure for eye examinations and suggested standards of vision for VDU operators. *Ophthal. Optician*, **December 8**, 50.

Association of Optometrists. *Statement of good practice for work with display screen equipment*. AOP, 233, Blackfriars Road, London.

Barfield, W. (1984). Stress as a function of increased cognitive load at a VDT. In *Ergonomics and health in modern offices. Proceedings of the International Conference, Turin, 7–November 1983.* (ed. E. Grandjean), pp. 181–6. Taylor and Francis Ltd, London.

Bauer, D., Bonacker, M., and Cavonius, C.R. (1983). Frame repetition rate for flicker free viewing of bright VDU screens. *Displays*, **January**, 31–2.

Bedwell, C.H. (1978). *Assessment of eye strain and difficulty in viewing visual display units*. Edited transcript of the one day meeting on eyestrain and VDUs, pp. 21–5. The Ergonomics Society, Loughborough, UK.

Bergquist, U.O.V. (1984). VDTS and health: a technical and medical appraisal of the state of art. *Scand. J. Work Environ. Health*, **10** (Suppl. 2), 1–87.

Birnbaum, R. (1978). *Health hazards of visual display units with particular reference to the office environment*. Review prepared for the Information and Advisory Service, TUC Centenary Institute of Occupational Health, London School of Hygiene and Tropical Medicine, London.

British College of Optometrists. *Work with display screen equipment*. Statement of good practice issued by the British College of Optometrists, 10, Knaresborough Place, London.

BS 7179 (1990) *Ergonomics of design and use of visual display terminals (VDTs) in offices*, Parts 1–6. BSI, London.

Cakir, A., Hart, D.J., and Stewart, T.F.M. (1980). *Visual display terminals*. John Wiley and Sons, Chichester.

Canadian Occupational Environmental Branch of the Ministry of Labour (1983). Working with visual display terminals. *Can. J. Optom.*, **45**, 134–40.

Chakman, J. and Guest, D.J. (1983). Vision and the visual display unit. A review. *Aust. J. Optom.*, **66**(4), 125–37.

CIBS (1984). *Code for interior lighting*. Chartered Institute for Building Services, London.

CIBSE (1989). *Lighting guide (LG3): Areas for visual display terminals.* Chartered Institute for Building Services, London.

Cole, B.L., Sharpe, K., Slack, A., and Maddocks, J.D. (1989). The Sec-VDU study. Comparison of refractive error and visual acuity of VDU users and non VDU users. *Bulletin No. 3*, Victorian College of Optometry, University of Melbourne, Australia.

Cox, E.A. (1980). *Radiation emissions from visual display units. Proceedings of the conference on health hazards of VDUs*, 1, p. 27. Loughborough University, Loughborough.

Cox, E.A. (1983). Electromagnetic radiation emissions from visual display units: a review. *Display Technology and Application*, **4**, 7–10.

Dain, S.J., McCarthy, A.K., and Chan-Ling, T. (1988). Symptoms in VDU operators. *Am. J. Optom. Physiol. Opt.*, **65**, 162–7.

Dainoff, M.J., Happ, A., and Crane, P. (1981). Visual fatigue and occupational stress in VDT operators. *Human Factors*, **23**, 421–38.

De Groot, J.P. and Kamphuis, A. (1983). Eye strain in VDU users: physical correlates and long-term effects. *Human Factors*, **25**, 409–13.

Display Screen Equipment work (1992). *Health and safety (display screen equipment) regulations 1992.* Guidance on Regulations L26, Health and Safety Executive, HMSO, London.

EC Directive (1990). Directive 90/270/EEC: the minimum safety and health requirements for work with display screen equipment. *Official Journal of the European Communities*, **L156**, 14–18.

Elliot, G., Gies, P., Joyner, K.H., and Roy, C.R. (1986). Electromagnetic radiation emissions from video display terminals (VDTs). *Clin. Exper. Optom.*, **69**(2), 53–61.

Fincham, E.F. (1951). The accommodation reflex and its stimulus. *Br. J. Ophthalmol.* **35**, 381–93.

Good, G.W. and Daum, K.M. (1985). *The use of progressive multifocals with video display terminals.* Ohio State University College of Optometry, Ohio.

Grundy, J.W. and Rosenthal, S.G. (1982). VDUs on site. *Ophthal. Optician*, **July 17**, 500.

Grundy, J.W., Rosenthal, S.G., and Seymour, H. (1991). *Visual aspects of VDU usage.* Association of Optometrists, 233–4, Blackfriars Road, London, SE1 8NW.

Gunnarsson, E. and Ostberg, O. (1977). *National Board of Occupational Safety and Health Reports 35: the physical and psychological working environment in a terminal-based computer storage and retrieval system.* Stockholm, Sweden.

Gunnarsson, E. and Soderberg, I. (1980). *Eye strain resulting from VDT work at the Swedish Telecommunication administration.* Stockholm National Board of Occupational Safety and Health. Stockholm, Sweden.

Hamard, H., Chevaleraud, J.P., Trubert, E., and Meillon, J.P. (1987). Presbyopic correction by use of progressive half spectacles among users of video terminals. *J. Fr. Ophthal.*, **10**, 505–13.

Health and Safety (Display Screen Equipment) Regulations (1992). No. 2792. HMSO, London.

Holler, H., Kundi, M., Schmid, H., Still, H.G., Thaler, A., and Winter, N. (1975). Arbeitsbeansprachung und Augenbelastung an Bildschirmgetaten Wein: Verlag des OGB. Cited by Mah, L.J. (1983). Aspects of visual stress in visual display terminal work. *Canad. J. Optom.* **45**, 124–7.

Horgen, G., Aaras, A., Fagerthun, H.E., and Larsen, S.E. (1989). The work posture and the postural load of the neck and shoulders when correcting presbyopia with different types of multifocal lenses on VDU-workers. In *Work with computers: organizational, management, stress and health aspects.* (ed. M.J. Smith and G. Salvendy). Elsevier Scientific Publishers B.V., Amsterdam.

HSE (1983). *Visual display units.* Health and Safety Executive, HMSO, London.

Hultgren, G.V. and Knave, B. (1974). Discomfort glare and disturbances from light reflections in an office landscape with CRT display terminals. *Appl. Ergonom.*, **5**, 2–8.

Knave, B. and Wideback, P.G. (1987). *Work with display units. 86.* Selected papers from the International Scientific Conference on work with display units. Stockholm, May 12–15 1986. Elsevier Science Publishers, Amsterdam.

Knave, B.G., Wibom, R.I., Hedstrom, L.D., and Bergquist, U.O.V. (1985). Work with video display terminals among office employees. 1. Subjective symptoms and discomfort. *Scand. J. Work. Environ. Health*, **11**, 457–66.

Laubli, T.H., Hünting, W., and Grandjean, E. (1980). Visual impairments in VDU operators related to environmental conditions. In *Ergonomic aspects of display terminals.* (ed. E. Grandjean and E. Vigliani), pp. 85–94.Taylor and Francis Ltd, London.

Levy, F. and Ramberg, I.G. (1987). Eye fatigue among VDU users and non-VDU users. In *Work with display units 86.* Selected papers from the International Scientific Conference on work with display units. Stockholm, May 12–15, 1986. (ed. B. Knave and P.G. Wideback) pp. 42–52. Elsevier Science Publishers, Amsterdam.

Marriott, I.A. and Stuchly, M.A. (1986). Health aspects of work with visual display terminals. *J. Occup. Med.*, **28**, 833–48.

Miller, S.C. (1984). Meeting the eye care needs of video display terminal operators. *J. Am. Optom. Assoc.*, **55**, 611–18.

Millodot, M. and Sivak, J. (1973). Influence of accommodation on the chromatic aberration of the eye. *Br. J. Physiol. Opt.*, **28**, 169–74.

Mousa, G.Y. (1986). Control of glare for VDT operators. 1. Transmission of fluorescent light through UV filters and pink lenses. *Can. J. Optom.*, **48**, 47–9.

Murch, G. (1982). How visible is your display? *Electro-Optical System Design*, **14**, 43–9.

NOISH (1981). *Potential health hazards of video display terminals.* Report No. 81–129. US Department of Health and Human Sciences, National Institute for Occupational Safety and Health, Cincinnati, Ohio.

Obstfeld, H. and Thomson, D. (1985). Visual display units, visual discomfort and VDU spectacles. *Optom. Today*, **November 9, 25**, 732–3.

Ong, C.N. and Phoon, W.O. (1987). Influence of age on performance and health of VDU workers. In *Work with display units 86.* Selected papers from the International Scientific Conference on work with display units. Stockholm, May 12–15 1986. (ed. B. Knave and P.G. Wideback), pp. 211–16. Elsevier Science Publishers, Amsterdam.

Osterberg, O. (1980). Accommodation and visual fatigue in display work. In *Ergonomic aspects of visual display terminals. Proceedings of the International Workshop, Milan, March 1980.* (ed. E. Grandjean and E. Vigliani), pp. 41–52. Taylor and Francis Ltd, London.

Phillips, S. and Stark, L. (1977). Blur: a sufficient accommodative stimulus. *Documenta Ophth.*, **3**, 65–89.

Reading, V. (1978). *Visual aspects and ergonomics of visual display units.* Institute of Ophthalmology, London.

Rey, P. and Meyer, J.J. (1980). Visual impairments and their objective correlates. In *Ergonomic aspects of visual display terminals. Proceedings of the International Workshop, Milan, March 1980.* (ed. E. Grandjean and E. Vigliani), pp. 77–83. Taylor and Francis Ltd, London.

Rosner, M. and Belkin, M. (1989). Video display units and visual function. *Surv. Ophthal.*, **33**, 515–22.

Rupp, B.A., McVey, B.W., and Taylor, S.E. (1984). Image quality and the accommodative response. In *Ergonomics and health in modern offices. Proceedings of the International Scientific Conference, Turin, November 7–9, 1983.* (ed. E. Grandjean), pp. 254–9. Taylor and Francis Ltd, London.

Rycroft, R.J.G. and Calnan, C.D. (1980). *Facial rashes among VDU operators. Proceedings of the Conference on the Health Hazards of VDUs 1*, p. 15. Loughborough University, UK.

Salvendy, G. (1982). Human computer communication with special reference to technology developments, occupational stress and educational needs. *Ergonomics*, **25**, 435–47.

Sauter, S.L. (1984). Preditors of strain in VDT users and traditional office workers. In *Ergonomics and health in modern offices. Proceedings of the International Scientific Conference, Turin, November 7–9, 1983.* (ed. E. Grandjean), pp. 129–35. Taylor and Francis Ltd, London.

Sivak, J.G. and Woo, G.C. (1983). Colour of visual display terminals and the eye. Green VDTs provide optimal stimulus to accommodation. *Am. J. Optom. Physiol. Opt.* **60**(7), 640–1.

Starr, S.J., Thompson, C.R., and Shute, S.J. (1982). Effects of video display terminals on telephone operators. *Human Factors*, **24**, 699–711.

Taylor, S.P. and Yeow, P.T. (1990). Visual display units—friend or foe? *The Optician*, **5234**, 18–22, **5237**, 19–23, **5241**, 15–19.

Terrana, T., Merluzzi, F., and Giudici, E. (1980). Electronic radiations emitted by visual display units. In *Ergonomic aspects of visual display terminals. Proceedings of the International Workshop, Milan, March 1980.* (ed. E. Grandjean and E. Vigliani), pp. 13–21. Taylor and Francis Ltd, London.

Tjonn, H.H. (1980). Report on facial rashes among operators in Norway. *Proceedings of the Conference on the health hazards of VDUs. 1*, pp. 19–23. Loughborough University. UK.

Ungar, P.E. (1971). Sight at work. *Work Study*, March, 46–8.

Varrall, G. (1983). The visual environment and new office technology. *Ophthal. Optician*, **June 4**, 401–4.

Weiss, M.M. and Peterson, R.C. (1979). Electromagnetic radiation emitted from video computer terminals. *Am. Ind. Hygiene. Assoc. J.*, **40**, 300–9.

Wilkins, A. (1978). *Epileptogenic attributes of TV and VDUs*. Edited transcript of the one day meeting on eyestrain and VDUs, pp. 27–35. The Ergonomics Society, Loughborough, UK.

Yekta, A.A., Jenkins, T., and Pickwell, D. (1987). The clinical assessment of binocular vision before and after a working day. *Ophthal. Physiol. Opt.*, **7**, 349–52.

Yeow, P.T. (1988). The effects of short term and long term VDU usage on visual functions and visual fatigue. PhD thesis, University of Wales.

Yeow, P.T. and Taylor, S.P. (1989). Effects of short term VDT usage on visual functions. *Optom. Vis. Sci.*, **66**, 459–66.

Further reading

Cakir, A., Hart, D.J., and Stewart, T.F.M. (1980). *Visual display terminals.* John Wiley and Sons, Chichester.

Grandjean, E. (ed.) (1984). *Ergonomics and health in modern offices.* Taylor and Francis Ltd, London, UK.

Grundy, J.W., Rosenthal, J.G., and Seymour, H. (1991). *Visual aspects of VDU usage*. The Association of Optometrists, 233–4, Blackfriars Road, London, SE1 8NW.

Pearce, B.G. (ed.) (1984). *Health hazards of VDTs?* John Wiley and Sons, Chichester.

Stewart, T.F.M. (1980). Problems caused by continuous use of visual display units. *Ltg. Res. Tech.*, **12**, 26–35.

10. Driving

Vision is the one human sense that is absolutely essential for safe driving. Although other senses relay important, but somewhat less essential, information to a driver, so that the appreciation of a situation is much improved, it is estimated that up to 90 per cent of the information received is visual. Clearly a blind person cannot be permitted to drive. However, as a person's vision can vary from blindness to 6/5, there must be a minimum standard below which it would be inadvisable for anyone to drive.

There has been a marked increase in the volume of traffic on the roads in recent years and the advances in car engine design mean that the traffic is now travelling at much higher speeds than before. Despite the increasing demands made on the driver of today, the visual standards required in the UK have remained virtually unchanged since they first came into operation in 1935. It may well be that in the present climate those standards are now inappropriate.

Surprisingly, there is very little evidence that relates the standard of vision to a driver's performance. Hence it is not easy to determine the minimum level of vision for safe driving. This situation also exists in other countries, as visual standards have never been internationally agreed. There are very obvious differences in the testing procedures and standards required by different countries. One of the simpler vision tests is used in the UK, involving only the reading of a number plate at a prescribed distance. In other countries, more rigorous examinations are used to assess visual functions, such as measurements of visual field, dark adaptation, stereopsis, and glare recovery.

Drivers need to cope with a wide range of confusing visual situations. For example, conditions when visibility is poor due to rain, mist, or fog, demand a good standard of vision for safe driving. Some studies have failed to relate poor vision to accident rate. This may be due to the fact that accidents do not generally have one single cause but often result from a combination of events. There are believed to be over 1000 independent factors affecting driver behaviour. These relate to the road conditions, the vehicle, and the driver. It is well understood that vision, fatigue, alcohol, vehicle visibility, road lighting, motor co-ordination, accident proneness, and attention affect a driver's behaviour. Fortunately, there is a certain amount of self-selection. Some people give up driving when their vision deteriorates to a level they consider unsafe. This is particularly evident amongst the elderly who 'do not like to drive at night' as they have reduced dark adaptation. They often restrict their driving to the daylight hours.

The UK injury/accident data for 1989 revealed 260 759 accidents, of which 185 871 occurred during daylight hours and 74 888 at night (Road Accidents Great Britain 1989). The total number of casualties involved in these accidents was 341 592. Although this number has increased since 1988, there has been a large increase in traffic and the casualty rate has in fact only increased by 1 per cent.

The TRRL (Transport and Road Research Laboratory) (1980) carried out a large study to identify the important factors that provoked accidents. They visited the site where the accident happened as soon as possible after the event and interviewed the driver at a later date (Staughton and Storie 1977). This 'on the spot' study investigated a total of 2036 accidents. The results of the study: showed that road user error was responsible for 95 per cent of the accidents and 44 per cent of the drivers at fault were judged to have made perceptual errors. The vehicle and road/environment were responsible for only 9 and 28 per cent of accidents, respectively. The perceptual errors made were mainly due to distraction and misjudgement of speed and distance. The latter is often due to a lack of visual adaptation to speed. After driving at 70 mph, 30 mph seems very slow, but to travel at 30 mph after being in a slow moving traffic jam seems relatively fast. The visual adaptation is believed to occur due to the streaming of the visual field across the periphery of the retina. A method of reducing accidents at roundabouts, where many accidents are due to drivers entering too fast, is to paint transverse bars across the road with decreasing separation. The lines are intended to create the illusion of speeding up if the driver continues to drive over them at a constant speed, and hence the driver will reduce speed. They also act as a visual hazard warning. These transverse bars have reduced accidents due to cars entering a roundabout too fast by about 60 per cent at 50 trial sites (Hills 1980).

Relationship between visual function and driving performance

Many studies have been carried out to try and relate visual abilities with driving performance (Burg 1967, 1968; Keeney 1968; Cashell 1970; Liesmaa 1973; Council and Allen 1974; Hills and Burg 1977; Hofstetter 1976).

Static visual acuity

Good central visual acuity and its associated clear retinal image is necessary for the early recognition and reading of road signs. It also aids the early detection of small and hazardous objects, such as pedestrians, motorcycles, and other obstacles in the roadway. Good acuity allows the driver more time to make decisions about events, obstacles, and signs and, in effect, slows down the action. A driver with poor acuity requires the obstacle to be closer before its significance can be appreciated, leaving less time to react. He or she must be more alert, will therefore fatigue faster and become more easily perceptually overloaded. For example, Allen (1969) states that someone with 6/6 vision driving at 60 mph has 3.9 s to read a road sign of 15 cm high (6-inch) letters; when the visual acuity is reduced to 6/12 there are only 1.95 s for this sign to be seen. This is reduced even further, to 0.78 s, when the acuity is 6/60.

Burg (1967, 1968) carried out one of the largest studies investigating the relationship between visual functions and driving ability. He assessed over 17 500 Californian drivers and compared their visual ability with their 3-year accident record. This study showed a weak, but statistically significant correlation between the vision scores and the driver accident rate. In 1977 this information was reanalysed with a view to establishing a new set of driver vision standards (Hills and Burg 1977). The sample, of well over 14 000 drivers, was subdivided into four age groups: (i) under 25 years; (ii) 25–39 years; (iii) 40–54; and (iv) over 54 years. It was found that static and dynamic visual acuity were the most important factors in the over 54-year-old age group, where there was a clear relationship between these factors and their accident rate.

However, the Road Research Laboratory (1963) analysed the results of four separate studies on drivers' vision and, suprisingly, concluded that the visual acuity has a relatively small, almost insignificant, correlation with accidents.

Liesmaa (1973) found a positive relationship between poor visual acuity and poor driving ability. He observed drivers' behaviour whilst overtaking or entering a major road, from an unmarked police car. Drivers considered to be dangerous were stopped and their monocular and binocular visual acuities were measured. The results obtained were then compared with a control group. In the group of people who were driving dangerously there were three times as many drivers who were monocular or who had visual acuities below the required level compared with the control group.

Hofstetter (1976) analysed the number of accidents and the visual acuities of 13 786 drivers. He found that, amongst those drivers who had been involved in three or more accidents, twice as many had poor acuity. The proportion in two accidents was about 50 per cent greater amongst the drivers with poor acuity. From this study it was not possible to determine a precise level of acuity at which a person could be considered safe to drive.

A recent report from Germany concluded that accidents did occur more frequently amongst drivers with considerably reduced photopic (daylight) vision, <6/9+ in one or both eyes, than those with adequate or slightly reduced vision (Hebenstreit 1984).

Several summaries of papers relating to visual ability and driving performance have been compiled. They have all come to the same conclusion: in general there is only a weak statistical association between static visual acuity and poor driving ability (Levitt 1975; Davison 1978; Hedin 1980).

Dynamic visual acuity

The strongest and most consistent relationship between the visual functions and the driving performance was found to be dynamic visual acuity (Burg 1967, 1968). This positive correlation indicates that good co-ordination and freedom from confusion and dizziness are very important when driving. Medical conditions that interfere with the vestibular mechanisms, such as Ménière's disease, or where there is a limitation of head movement, such as in arthritis, can affect the dynamic visual acuity. A reduction of dynamic visual acuity will also occur if the static visual acuity is defective. Burg's data (1967, 1968) were reanalysed by Hills and Burg (1977), who found that only the older age group (over 54 years) show a consistent relationship between dynamic visual acuity and accident rate.

Colour vision

Various studies have been carried out to determine the relationship between the accident rate and colour vision defects. Norman (1960) studied a number of London bus drivers, but did not find a higher accident rate or traffic violation rate in 149 colour defective drivers than in the control group of 149 drivers who had normal colour vision.

Colour vision defects may be hazardous if they cause confusion between the red, green, and amber signal lights. According to Coles and Brown (1966) a protanope (red colour-blind) requires about four times the normal intensity to see a red light. People with red colour vision defects may also find it difficult when driving in fog, or at night, as they are unable to fully appreciate a red tail/brake light. It would be advisable for them not to wear tinted spectacles when driving as these reduce/modify the amount of light reaching the eyes.

Peripheral visual fields

With such a high volume of traffic on the roads today, good peripheral vision is essential. A restriction of the visual field can never be fully overcome although increasing head and eye movements and adding extra mirrors to the car can be of help. The visual field is important for maintaining the driver's orientation and in establishing relationships between the many objects in the field of view. Central vision, important as it is, can only fixate the pavement once every 7 m (22 ft) at 95 km/h 60 mph. The remaining portions of the roadway between and to the left and right of the fixations must be taken in by peripheral vision (Allen 1969).

There have been varied reports concerning the relationship between visual field defects and accident rate. A review of the studies was made by North (1985). A few of the reports showing a positive correlation, follow:

Johnson and Keltner (1983) screened 10 000 drivers and compared their driving record over the previous 3 years with their visual field. They found that drivers with binocular visual field loss had accident and conviction rates that were twice as high as those of a control group.

Kite and King (1961) found that a gross reduction of visual field on one side or monocularity, is associated with seven-fold increases in crashes at road intersections and pedestrian injuries.

Keeney (1968) noted that monocular drivers were four times more likely to be found amongst those cited for multiple driving violations (80 out of 991) than to be found in an ophthalmic practice patient population (424 of 21 000).

It would appear from the above research that visual field defects are related to accidents. Keeney (1968) suggests that a visual field of 140 ° is advisable for driving and defensible in court as a minimum standard. This standard can be met by a monocular person, but it is important to note that a driver who becomes monocular, perhaps due to an eye injury, should be allowed time to adapt to the loss of visual field, reduced depth perception, and the effect of the blind spot (which produces an absolute scotoma within the visual field). In Sweden, a driver is banned for 1 year after the loss of vision in an eye.

No evidence was found by Hills and Burg (1977), or by Council and Allen (1974), to support the 140 ° visual standard proposed. Council and Allen (1974) studied the driving performance and visual fields of 52 000 North Carolina drivers. They concluded that, overall, the 2-year accident records of drivers with limited visual fields (< 140 °) were no different from those with normal visual fields (> 160 °). They did find that re- stricted visual fields may be slightly related to a higher proportion of side collisions, but overall these drivers had no higher accident rate.

Visual fields can be artificially reduced, for example by aphakic spec- tacle corrections, thick spectacle frames and sides, and by car design. There are obvious pathological disorders that can also cause visual defects, such as glaucoma, retinitis pigmentosa, and cataracts. Elkington and MacKean (1982) studied 214 patients suffering from open-angle glaucoma. They found that many of them experienced difficulty when driving and, in six cases, glaucoma was diagnosed as a result of the patient becoming aware of a visual field defect whilst driving. Of the patients who were still driving (61 out of the 214), only five were aware of their visual field defect and made allowances for it by head movements. This report was concluded by raising the question as to the duty of medical practitioners to advise their patients when they are considered to be unsafe to drive due to their visual field loss.

Stereopsis and oculomotor balance

Stereoscopic vision is the ability to appreciate depth by the superimposi- tion of two slightly dissimilar objects. The position of objects can be located with one eye by monocular cues such as relative size, position relative to the horizontal, contrast, movement, brightness, etc. Unfortu- nately, under conditions of poor visibility, e.g. at night, the majority of the monocular cues are missing and stereopsis becomes the major cue in depth perception. Stereopsis is inoperative beyond 500 m and therefore of little benefit in high speed driving, although it is valuable for nearer tasks, such as parking a car or locating children around cars, buses, etc. (Allen 1969).

It seems that stereopsis is not related to safe driving, as no correlation has been found between defective stereoscopic vision and increased accident frequency (Burg 1968). Keeney (1968) states that stereoscopic vision is not important for the distances found in traffic.

The absence of stereopsis can be due to a squint. The presence of a squint without double vision is no obstacle to driving because the peripheral visual field is normal. However, the presence of double vision does constitute an obstacle to driving.

A horizontal phoria, although known to be enhanced by fatigue, low illumination, and alcohol, has not been shown to correlate with crash rate (Burg, 1967). However, a vertical phoria of greater than 1 prism dioptre was found to be associated with poor accident records, especially in the over 55-year-olds (Davison 1985).

Night vision

It is often found that the accident rate relative to distance travelled during the hours of darkness, is greater than that during the hours of daylight. Accidents occuring at night are also more likely to result in fatalities or severe injuries, and the majority of accidents to pedestrians occur at night. The increase of potential accidents during the hours of darkness is partly due to poor street lighting and to the glare from oncoming headlights reducing visibility.

Studies by Allen (1969) have shown that night vision performance, measured by the ability to detect objects at night in a laboratory and a field situation, can be severely handicapped by a refractive error. A driver with 6/12 day acuity was found to require 5 to 100 times more illumination to detect a given target than he would have required if he had a day time acuity of 6/6. This means that 6/12 by day cuts the critical perception distance in half compared with 6/6. At night it may cut it to one-tenth or less. Therefore, Allen suggests that drivers with a daytime visual acuity of 6/12, should not be permitted to drive at night at all.

Static visual acuity, or contrast sensitivity, testing under night driving conditions is urgently needed according to Hedin (1980), who also suggests alterations to the regulations to allow the issue of a driver's licence valid only during daylight hours if deemed necessary.

Night myopia

A phenomenon known as night myopia may also influence night driving. People become relatively more short-sighted at night. This myopic shift can be as much as 4 D (Leibowitz and Owens 1978), although it varies from person to person and with the level of lighting. There may be quite marked short-term variations and the dark focus can also be affected by non-visual factors such as psychological stress (Hope and Rubin 1984). Hence, there are problems in prescribing spectacles for night driving: (i) several refractions on different days may be required to determine the representative dark focus to take into account patient variability; and (ii) the prescription found will be appropriate only for a limited set of conditions.

The Association of Optometrists (1990) has made a statement about night myopia and prescribing a correction. It suggests that the variable nature of the myopia induced at low levels of illumination creates a major problem in prescribing a correction. When driving at night there is never total darkness, as there is light from car headlights, street lamps, etc. Under conditions of low illumination (mesopic level) the degree of myopia induced will be reduced and, as stated, it will vary according to the lighting level so that a single prescription will not be suitable. Also, if a correction is provided there may be problems for the driver when travelling into a well lit area. The extra negative power of the correction may become a hazard because it may induce confusion, misjudgement of distances, and speeds, etc. The difficulties encountered by a driver at night are not just due to myopia; there are other factors, such as increased reaction time and increased glare recovery time. Therefore, the provision of a correction is not a simple answer to the difficulties experienced by many when driving at night.

Another possible reason for the high rate of road traffic accidents at night is that drivers appear to be less cautious. This was demonstrated when drivers were observed turning at a T-junction on to the main road. In the daylight most drivers waited for gaps of 6.5–7.5 s before pulling out, whereas at night they pulled out after gaps of only 3.5–5.5 s. Drivers, therefore, incurred a much higher risk of being involved in a collision. It is believed that there is a 40 per cent greater chance of collision on a busy T-junction at night because of the willingness of emerging vehicles to go for shorter gaps, and it is 12 times more likely that the collision will be serious (Transport and Road Research Laboratory, 1980).

Glare

Many drivers complain about glare during night driving. It is due mainly to dirt and scratches on the windscreen causing scattering of light. Smoke from cigarettes can cause an increase in glare from oncoming headlights at night and will cause veiling glare during the day. Allen (1969) estimates that windscreens should be replaced every 50 000 miles due to wear and tear. Tinted windscreens and the use of tinted spectacles are detrimental to those visual functions that are important for night driving:

(1) glare recovery, i.e. speed of retinal recovery after being dazzled by glare;

(2) glare resistance, i.e. the ability to see against glare;

(3) visual acuity, i.e. the ability to see efficiently in low illumination.

GLARE RECOVERY

The recovery time of retinal sensitivity not only increases with age but also with the use of tinted spectacles or windscreens, and the level of dark adaptation. Many elderly patients wear tinted spectacles to reduce the amount of light entering the eye, and thereby reduce the light scattering. Research shows that it takes longer to recover from glare when using tints. Although drivers feel more comfortable visually, tinted lenses do not improve performance. Phillips and Rutstein (1965) found that glare recovery increased by an average of 54 per cent, from 2.03 s to 3.02 s, with tinted spectacles. The colour of the tint is irrelevant, as the increase of retinal sensitivity depends upon the absorption of the lenses.

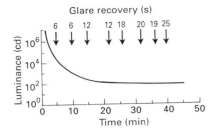

Glare recovery (s)

Fig. 10.1 The influence of dark adaptation upon glare recovery. The curve represents the normal course of dark adaptation. It can be seen that the glare recovery time after dazzle, i.e. the time for readaptation, increases with duration of dark adaptation (after Papst 1962, courtesy of the *New Scientist*).

Tinted lenses increase the time required for dark adaptation (Davey and Sheridan 1953; McFarland *et al.* 1960; Wolf *et al.* 1960). The time for readaptation also increases with increasing dark adaptation. For example, the recovery from glare took 6 s and 25 s after 5 and 38 min of dark adaptation, respectively (Papst 1962; Fig. 10.1).

Glare resistance
This is the ability to see against glare. Visual recovery time during glare increase by about 25 per cent when wearing tinted spectacles (Davey 1959; Phillips and Rutstein 1967).

Visual acuity
Tinted spectacles reduce the visual acuity during day and night driving conditions (Richards 1953; Wolf *et al.* 1960). Visual acuity is found to decrease in proportion to the reduction in transmission of light and is not affected by the colour of the tint (Sturgis and Osgood 1982).

Yellow night driving glasses are popular because they reduce glare. However, although the tint does diminish the amount of light entering the eye, and so reduces glare, other areas of the visual field can be covered with a dangerous level of darkness; their use is not recommended. They give the subjective impression of brightening the overall scene whilst, in fact, reducing the contrast of objects against an already dark background. Similarly, tinted windscreens are also detrimental to visual functions and are not recommended for night driving (Wolf *et al.* 1960).

There are several theories as to the subjective preference for yellow tints (Phillips and Rutstein 1965):

1. Yellow is associated with the high luminous efficiency of sodium lamps and, hence, implies good vision.
2. Glare is reduced by yellow headlights in foggy conditions. However, the reduction in glare is not due to the colour, but to the reduced intensity.
3. There is less glare from the yellow car headlamps used in France, but this is mainly due to the sharply cut-off beam pattern.
4. Yellow is associated with sunlight and a subjective impression of increased luminance.

No driver should wear tinted spectacles at night because of the reduction in visual function, which is further reduced by tinted or dirty windscreens and by age.

There is no real necessity to have a tinted windscreen. Although drivers will argue that their vision is more comfortable with the tint during the daytime, there is a potential night-time hazard caused by loss of light transmission. Even the angle at which the windscreen is mounted can reduce the amount of light transmitted. Most are at an angle of 60 °, which, apart from making it an ideal dirt collector, will cause a 20 per cent loss of transmission due to reflection. A tinted windscreen is also supposed to absorb heat and reduce glare. However, it is is very inefficient in performing both of these functions; only 25 per cent of solar heat is absorbed. It would be better to paint the car in light colours and insulate the roof and floor, as this would reduce the heat by about 44 per cent (Allen 1969). It should also be noted that there is not enough reduction in transmission of light to help reduce glare on a bright day. In bright conditions it would be better to wear tinted spectacles.

There are ways of reducing the number of road traffic accidents that occur at night. One survey (Sabey and Johnson 1973) analysed the relationship between night-time accidents and street lighting and found a considerable reduction in the number of accidents when street lighting was improved. Improving the standard of street lighting on trunk roads reduces the number of accidents and saves money, despite the cost of installation. An estimate of the saving in the cost of accidents on roads where a 70 mph speed limit applies was about three times the annual cost of the lighting. It appears that, in addition to reducing the number of road traffic accidents, the crime rate is reduced.

Road lighting is designed to provide a bright visual background against which drivers see a potential hazard as a dark silhouette. On a well lit road the use of dipped headlights does not generally help drivers themselves for the following reasons:

(1) dipped headlights act as a glare source to all road users;
(2) pedestrians and drivers can be dazzled by them;
(3) the silhouette contrast is decreased which, in turn, reduces the visibility of hazards, etc.

One advantage of a dipped beam is that road users are aware of the presence of a moving vehicle. The use of side lights overcomes the problems of glare and reduced contrast but they are so dim (one-hundredth the brightness of a dipped beam) that the vehicle is very difficult to detect. A solution to this problem has been proposed by the Department of Transport, which has suggested fitting a 'dim-dip' lighting device to a dipped-beam headlamp. This should result in the emission of a beam of an intensity of between 10 and 20 per cent of the intensity of the normal dipped beam. It should provide glare-free lighting and allow the vehicle to be detected (Road Vehicle Lighting Regulations 1989).

Other factors

Alcohol

Alcohol impairs mental efficiency, acts as an anaesthetic, and slows the response to a hazardous situation. It also can cause diplopia and blurring of vision. Moreover, the effects of smoking are summative with the effects of alcohol.

The legislation making it an offence to drive with over 80 mg of alcohol/100 ml of blood was introduced in 1967 and had a marked effect on the number of road casualties. Figure 10.2 shows the total number of casualties (fatal, seriously, and slightly injured) in accidents involving illegal alcohol levels (Road Accidents Great Britain 1989); there has been a progressive reduction. The 20–29 age group has the highest percentage of fatalities due to illegal alcohol levels. However, there is an encouraging downward trend in the younger age groups in drink-drive accidents. Whilst these findings are encouraging, drinking and driving is still a

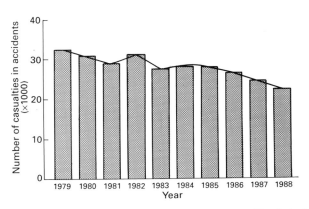

Fig. 10.2 Estimates of total casualties in accidents involving illegal alcohol levels (adjusted for under reporting, after Road Accidents Great Britain 1989).

serious problem. It is estimated that, in 1988, one in six of deaths and one serious injury in eleven was associated with illegal alcohol levels (Road Accidents Great Britain 1989).

Age

As mentioned, visual functions change with age. There are changes in visual acuity, contrast sensitivity, visual fields, glare sensitivity, and other visual capabilities. Many eye disorders that cause a reduction in visual acuity or visual fields are prevalent amongst the elderly, e.g. cataracts, open angle glaucoma, and macular degeneration. Therefore, one might expect to find a higher accident rate amongst the elderly. However, a higher accident rate may not be due primarily to poor vision, but to other factors. Burg (1975) found that accidents occur more frequent in drivers < 25 and > 54 years of age. There is little difference between the accident rates for males and females. Accidents occuring to younger drivers who had good vision may have been due to inexperience, reckless driving, or alcohol abuse. Older drivers may have poorer vision but there are other factors, such as slower reaction times and duller hearing which confuse their assessment. As a result Burg suggests that poor vision can not be stated as being the major cause of accidents in the elderly, and improving their visual performance will not necessarily improve the accident rate. Figures from Road Accidents Great Britain (1989) of the number of casualties in various age groups do not appear to show a higher number of accidents occuring to the older age group. However, it is difficult to compare these results as the age groups selected are different (Fig. 10.3).

Rackhoff and Mourant (1979) investigated the eye movements of a group of young drivers (21–29 years) and a group of older drivers (46–60 years). They found that the older drivers made longer eye movements during a car-following task. One explanation for this is that older drivers have poorer parafoveal vision and so have to fixate foveally to acquire information, whereas younger drivers use their peripheral vision to gain

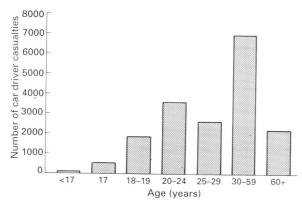

Fig. 10.3 Number of car driver casualties (killed or seriously injured) according to age (after Road Accidents Great Britain 1989).

the necessary information. Older drivers were found to have longer eye open times, which is presumably due to the fact that they need more time to acquire the relevant information. The ability to select relevant visual stimuli from an environment full of other distracting stimuli is impaired with age. This is an important factor in such tasks as driving, when the ability to select the relevant information quickly is necessary to avoid dangerous situations and accidents (Kahneman *et al.* 1973; Mihal and Barrett 1976).

Several surveys confirm the belief that older drivers travel at slower speeds and that they try to restrict their driving to low stress environments by, for example, avoiding driving at night or on icy roads (Case *et al.* 1970; Rackhoff 1974). However, despite this, accident rates for failing to give right of way, improper turning, or ignoring stop signs are higher for older drivers than for the middle-aged (McFarland *et al.* 1964; Keltner and Johnson 1987).

Keltner and Johnson (1987) conducted a survey of the Department of Motor Vehicles in 50 American states, studying the accident and conviction rates for different age groups. They found that although the elderly were responsible for a small percentage of traffic accidents, the type of accident in which they were involved could be related to peripheral and central visual field problems, e.g. intersection collisions, failure to yield right of way. They concluded that, as age-related changes in visual functions occur at different rates for different people, licensing of the elderly should be based on functional abilities rather than age. Therefore, they suggested that evaluation of visual acuity and visual fields should be performed every one to two years in those drivers over 65 years of age.

Summary

Many studies have failed to show that poor vision is an important cause of accidents. Burg (1967) points out the following difficulties in trying to relate driving performance to visual capabilities:

1. Vision is only one of many factors influencing driving performance.
2. There may be disparity between the visual capabilities and the degree to which they are used when driving.
3. Tests used may measure characteristics that are not closely related to the visual requirements of driving.
4. Reliability of criteria used to measure driving performance may be low.
5. Research methods may have short-comings, such as an unrepresentative sample of the driving population.

Spectacles for vehicle drivers

In this section I would like to make a number of points regarding the dispensing of spectacles for motorists.

First, the frame should have thin rims and sides, so that it does not restrict peripheral vision. The eye size chosen should be as large as possible, bearing in mind the prescription, again to allow the widest field of view. Lenses should be impact resistant, i.e. either plastics or toughened lenses should be used. If bifocals are required they should be dispensed with the smallest bifocal segment for driving spectacles. This is not to say that Executive bifocals are unsafe, after all, many people wear them when driving without any problems, but they may not be ideal. Any bifocal or trifocal lens must be dispensed so that the reading portion does not encroach on the distance vision, i.e. fit the segment top low (Bateman 1986). Varifocals do not appear to be a problem for drivers if they are correctly dispensed. In fact, many drivers find them very useful when parking, as they can see the car bonnet clearly through the intermediate portion of the lens.

Ideally, tinted spectacles should not be worn for night driving, unless they are proven to be clinically necessary, nor should they be worn in conditions of poor visibility.

Tinted lenses for daytime driving may be considered under the following headings:

1. *Photochromics*. These do not work very well in vehicles as the UV light that activates them is absorbed by the windscreen and windows of the car. Heat also lightens the lenses. Hence, the lenses will not darken to their full potential inside a warm vehicle. They are most frequently made of glass, although plastics are available. Photochromics perform better than uncoated white crown glass by day but are worse at night (Allen 1979).

2. *Polarizing lenses*. These are particularly effective in reducing the glare from the road surface when driving towards the sun. They give the greatest benefit in the evening and winter months, when the sun is low and the roads may be wet. However, problems may arise if the driver has a toughened glass windscreen or Triplex laminated glass, as the strain pattern will be clearly visible. Some drivers do not object to this pattern but others do not like it. Polarizing lenses are often

thought to absorb the UV/blue end of the spectrum. However, this is not necessarily true.

3. *UV/blue-absorbing lenses*. These lenses absorbing wavelengths up to 500 nm are useful for drivers. UV light is important because it causes fluorescence of the crystalline lens proteins. The visible light produced is then scattered over the retinal surface and reduces visibility. Examples of UV-absorbing lenses are UV 400, UVPLS 530, 540, 550 from Norville, Essilor's UVX coating or Zeiss Clarlets with Super ET coating.

A driver who wears sun spectacles with a deep tint is relatively more dark-adapted than the driver without sun spectacles. This means that if the sun spectacles are removed on entering a tunnel the driver will be able to see more clearly than the more light-adapted driver (Davey 1974).

There is a British Standard (BS 4110 1979), which recommends various types of impact resistant eye protectors for vehicle users, including visors, goggles, and spectacles. It also states the transmission of the lenses and the minimum field of vision that should be present when wearing an eye protector.

Visual standards for driving licences

National Standards for private motorists

Since 1935 it has been necessary for drivers of private vehicles in the UK to satisfy a minimum visual standard.

The licence application form (DVLA 1990) asks 'Is there anything wrong with your eyesight, such as double vision, tunnel vision, partial loss of sight, or night blindness?'

A booklet, *The medical aspects of fitness to drive*, has been published by the Medical Commission on Accident Prevention to give guidance to medical practitioners. Briefly the recommendations suggest, regarding vision, that drivers with double vision are considered unfit to drive unless the diplopia can be overcome by a prismatic correction. Binocular field defects such as bitemporal hemianopia or homonymous hemianopia, if complete or substantial in the lower quadrants, are a bar to driving. A binocular visual field of less than 120 degrees is considered unsafe. A driver with one eye may drive providing the visual field is full. However, the recent loss of an eye may require a short adaptation period.

Guidelines have been issued by the DVLC as to the parameters needed for the different types of field testing equipment used (Munton 1988).

In the UK, the Council of the Faculty of Ophthalmologists has recommended that the minimum visual field for safe driving could be defined as a field of vision of at least 120 degrees along the horizontal and of at least 20 degrees above and below the horizontal, measured by perimetry using a 3 mm white test object at 0.33 m (or equivalent perimeter).

In the UK all drivers must also meet the requirements of general statutes, which provide that drivers must be 'fit' and not likely to be a source of danger to the public. The application form (DVLA D1 1990) lists various medical conditions that should be declared: limb disability, epilepsy or fits, diabetes, multiple sclerosis, Parkinson's disease, sudden attacks of disabling giddiness or fainting, mental illness, disorder or disability, stroke(s), alcohol or drug abuse problem, heart pain recurring at rest, use of a cardiac pacemaker, and any kind of brain surgery should be reported. Drivers who suffer from insulin-dependent diabetes need to have their licence renewed every 3 years, when medical evidence will be required to support its renewal. Recent changes in legislation allow those diabetics treated by diet alone to hold the usual licence.

Drivers are required to read a number plate in good daylight (with glasses or contact lenses if worn) containing letters and figures 79.4 mm high at a distance of 20.5 m (Statutory Instrument No. 1378 1987). These symbols subtend a visual angle of 31.4 min of arc at the eye. The number-plate test is not considered to be a good test. One major point of criticism is that test conditions are poorly controlled, e.g. lighting, distance, and type and cleanliness of number plate. The standard of visual acuity required to read the number plate is greater than the nominal Snellen equivalent of 6/15. On examination of those who failed the number plate test, it was found to be equivalent to a clinical Snellen value of about 6/9−2 (Drasdo and Haggerty 1981). The number-plate test is often considered to be irrelevant to the driving situation, as it is a static test in good daylight. Other tests of visual competence should be checked, such as visual field, dynamic visual acuity, and contrast sensitivity.

The test is carried out at the time of the driving examination and is not repeated until the age of 70 years. It has been suggested recently that drivers applying for a provisional licence should be tested and drivers over 50 years of age should be examined at regular intervals. At present the driving licence is valid until the age of 70 years, with renewal every 3 years thereafter. Most people are not good at assessing whether their vision is up to standard, which was one reason why a number plate was used, to enable self-checking. However, various studies show an alarmingly high percentage of drivers who are ignorant of the visual standard required. A survey by the Optical Information Council (1979) showed that 56 percent of drivers, when asked the distance of the number-plate test, either did not know or gave the wrong answer. A similar figure of 59 per cent for the same question was reported by McCaghrey (1986). Another survey by Guest and Jennings (1983) showed that 12 per cent of drivers fail to meet the driving standard test. The findings of Davison and Irving (1980) regarding the decline of visual acuity with age also supports the need for regular re-checks amongst the older driving population.

Large goods and passenger-carrying vehicles licence

On 1 April 1991 the system that provided separate licences for drivers of cars, lorries, and buses ceased and a single licence is now issued, which shows the driving entitlement. This change brings the UK into line with other members of the EC. Drivers still need to pass separate tests and meet higher medical standards before they can drive lorries and buses. The terms 'heavy goods vehicle' (HGV) and 'public service vehicle' (PSV) have been renamed 'Large Goods Vehicle' (LGV) and

'Passenger Carrying Vehicle' (PCV), respectively. These vocational driving licences are issued or renewed from the Driver and Vehicle Licensing Centre at Swansea, although duplicates of the old style HGV and PSV licences that have been lost or destroyed, can still be issued by the Traffic Commissioners.

The publication *Driver licensing for lorries and buses in the 1990s*, DVLA states the health standards necessary. The eye sight standards require new drivers to have a visual acuity of not less than 6/9 in the better eye and not less than 6/12 in the other eye, with corrective lenses, including contact lenses, if worn. They must also meet an uncorrected standard of not less than 3/60 in each eye. All drivers who have monocular vision, diplopia, defective binocular vision, or visual field defects should be regarded as unfit to drive LCV or PCVs. Existing licence holders who obtained a licence before 1 January 1983 and who still held one on 1 April 1991, are allowed a concession to meet the earlier standard of not less than 6/12 in the better eye and not less than 6/36 in the other eye. If drivers need to wear glasses or contact lenses they must have an uncorrected acuity in each eye of not less than 3/60. The uncorrected standard of vision (3/60) effectively precludes from driving those who have had a cataract removed from one or both eyes, unless an intra-ocular lens has been inserted. The licence is valid up to the age of 45, or for 5 years, whichever is longer. From the age of 45 renewals are required every 5 years and, from the age of 65, annually.

The driver also has to pass a general medical examination before being declared fit to drive. Some of the conditions that make it unsafe to drive are: disorders of the heart, circulation, brain and nervous system; mental illness; and addiction to alcohol and drugs. A vocational licence will not be granted to an applicant who has suffered from an epileptic attack after the age of five or to insulin-dependent diabetics, although an exception is made for those insulin-dependent diabetics who held a valid licence on 1 April 1991, provided the Traffic Commissioner who issued it had knowledge of the condition before that date. (For further details refer to the Medical Commission on Accident Prevention 1985.)

Drivers are also required to inform the Drivers Medical Branch, DVLC, Swansea SA99 1TU, if any illness or disability develops or worsens, unless (like a sprained ankle) it is likely to get better within 3 months.

Any medical practitioner who is in any doubt about the advice that should given a patient about fitness to drive in any particular case, can discuss the matter with the Medical Adviser to the Department of Transport.

Summary

This chapter has attempted to show how difficult it is to set standards of vision associated with safe driving and suggests that other factors, such as driver education, should also be assessed and that street and vehicle lighting should be improved. Charman (1986) suggests that changing drivers' attitudes through education is the simplest way to reduce accidents. For example, the average driver's behaviour and road speed apparently change very little, regardless of the time of day and the level of visibility. It is estimated that total cost of road accidents in 1989 in the UK was £6 360 million, and the average cost per casualty was £13 290 (Road Accidents Great Britain 1989). Although it will be expensive to provide education for drivers and improve road and vehicle lighting, the cost in human suffering and the estimated cost of road traffic accidents, must be taken into account.

References

Allen, M.J. (1969). Vision and driving. *Traff. Saf. Res. Rev.*, **8**, 8–11.

Allen, M.J. (1979). Highway tests of photochromic lenses. *J. Am. Optom. Assoc.*, **59**, 1023–7.

Association of Optometrists (1990). AOP statement on night myopia. *Optom. Today*, **November 19**, 13, 19.

Bateman, N.F. (1986). Dispensing to car drivers. *Disp. Opt.*, **March**, 28.

BS 4110 (1979). *Eye-protectors for vehicle users. Amendments: 4630, July 1984 and 5890, April 1989*. BSI, London.

Burg, A. (1967). *The relationship between vision test scores and driving record: general findings. Report 62–74*. University of California, Los Angeles.

Burg, A. (1968). *Vision test scores and driving record: additional findings. Report 68–21*. University of California, Los Angeles.

Burg, A. (1975). The relationship between visual ability and road accidents. In *Prevention Routiere Internationale, First International Congress on Vision and Road Safety, Paris, 3–12*.

Case, H.W., Hulbert, S., and Beers, J. (1970). *Driving ability as affected by age. Final Report No. 70–18*. Institute of Transportation and Traffic Engineering, University of California, Los Angeles.

Cashell, G.T.W. (1970). Visual functions in relation to road accidents. *Injury*, **2**, 9–10.

Charman, W.N. (1985). Visual standards for driving. *Ophthal. Physiol. Opt.*, **5**, 211–20.

Charman, W.N. (1986). Vision and driving. *The Optician*, **192**, 27–32.

Coles, B.L. and Brown, B. (1966). Optimum intensity of red road-traffic signal lights for normal and protanopic observers. *J. Optom. Soc. Am.*, **56**, 516–22.

Council, F.M. and Allen, J.A. (1974). A study of the visual fields of North Carolina drivers and their relationship to accidents. Highway Research Safety Centre, University of North Carolina.

Davey, J.B. (1959). Seeing times with yellow glasses—a preliminary report. *The Optician*, **136**, 651.

Davey, J.B. (1974). Sunspectacles for drivers. *Ophthal. Optician*, **March 2**, 154–67.

Davey, J.B. and Sheridan, M. (1953). Night driving spectacles and night vision. *The Optician*, **July 31**, 33–8.

Davison, P.A. (1978). The role of drivers' vision in road safety. *Ltg. Res. Tech.*, **10**, 125–39.

Davison, P.A. (1985). Inter-relationships between British driver's ability, visual abilities, age and road accident histories. *Ophthal. Physiol. Opt.*, **5**, 195–204.

Davison, P.A. and Irving, A. (1980). *Survey of visual acuity of drivers. Transport and Road Research Laboratory Report No. 945*. Transport and Road Research Laboratory, Crowthorne, Berkshire.

Department of Transport (1985). *Road Accidents GB, 1984*. HMSO, London.

Drasdo, N. and Haggerty, C.M. (1981). A comparison of British number plate and Snellen vision tests for car drivers. *Ophthal. Physiol. Opt.*, 1, 39–54.

DVLA (1990). *Driver licensing for buses* and *lorries in the 1990s*, D200, section E, p. 7. HMSO, London.

DVLA (1990). Application for driving licence, D1 April, section 5 and 6., HMSO, London.

Elkington, A.R. and MacKean, J.M. (1982). Glaucoma and driving. *Br. Med. J.*, 285, 777–8.

Guest, D.J. and Jennings, J.B. (1983). A survey of drivers vision in Victoria. *Aust. J. Optom.*, 66, 13–19.

Hebenstreit, B.V. (1984). Visual acuity and road accidents (Sehvermogen und verkehrsunfalle). *Klin. Montsbl. Augenheilk.*, 185, 86–90.

Hedin, A. (1980). Retesting of vehicle drivers' visual capacity. *J. Traff. Med.*, 8, 18–21.

Hills, B.L. (1980). Vision, visibility and perception in driving. *Perception*, 9, 183–216.

Hills, B.L. and Burg, A. (1977). *A reanalysis of California driver vision data: general findings. Transport and Road Research Laboratory, Report No. LR768.* Transport and Road Research Laboratory, Crowthorne, Berkshire.

Hofstetter, H.W. (1976). Visual acuity and highway accidents. *J. Am. Optom. Assoc.*, 47, 887–93.

Hope, G.M. and Rubin, M.L. (1984). Perspectives in refraction: night myopia. *Surv. Ophthal.*, 29, 129–36.

Johnson, C.A. and Keltner, J.L. (1983). Incidence of visual field loss in 20 000 eyes and its relationship to driving performance. *Arch. Ophthalmol.*, 101, 371–5.

Kahneman, D., Ben-Ishai, R., and Lotan, M. (1973). Relation of a test of attention to road accidents. *J. Appl. Psychol.*, 58, 113–15.

Keltner, J.L. and Johnson, C.A. (1987). Visual function, driving safety and the elderly. *Ophthalmology*, 94, 1180–8.

Keeney, A.H. (1968). Relationship of ocular pathology and driving impairment. *Trans. Am. Acad. Ophthal. Otol.*, 72, 737–40.

Kite, C.R. and King, J.N. (1961). A survey of the factors limiting the visual fields of motor vehicle drivers in relation to minimum visual field and visibility standards. *Br. J. Physiol.*, 18, 85–107.

Leibowitz, H.W. and Owens, D.A. (1978). New evidence for the intermediate position of relaxed accommodation. *Documenta Ophth.*, 46, 133–47.

Levitt, J.G. (1975). Vision and driving. *Ophthal. Optician*, **December 13**, 1109–16.

Liesmaa, M. (1973). The influence of drivers' vision in relation to his driving. *The Optician*, 166, 10–13.

McCaghrey, G.E. (1986). Vision and driving. Motorfair Survey, 1985. *Optom. Today*, **March 1**, 132–6.

McFarland, R., Domey, R.G., Warren, A.B., and Ward, D.C. (1960). Dark adaptation as a function of age: I. A statistical analysis. *J. Gerontol.*, 15, 149–54.

McFarland, R.A., Tune, G.S., and Welford, A.T. (1964). On the driving of automobiles by older people. *J. Gerontol.*, 19, 190–7.

Medical Commission on Accident Prevention (1985). *Medical aspects of fitness to drive—a guide for medical practitioners*, (5th edn). The Medical Commission on Accident Prevention, 35–43 Lincoln's Inn Fields, London.

Mihal, W.L. and Barret, G.V. (1976). Individual differences in perceptual information processing and their relation to automobile accident involvement. *J. Appl. Psychol.*, 61, 229–33.

Munton, G. (1988). Form CLE 1060. DVLC Drivers Medical Branch.

Norman, L.G. (1960). Medical aspects of road safety. *Lancet*, **1**, 989–94, 1039–45.

North, R.V. (1985). The relationship between the extent of the visual field and driving performance. *Ophthal. Physiol.* Opt., **5**, 205–10.

Optical Information Council (1979). *Attitudes to eye care.* Optical Information Council, Temple Chambers, Temple Ave, London.

Papst, W. (1962). Dazzle and night driving. *New Scientist*, **314**, 436–8.

Phillips, A.J. and Rutstein, A. (1965). Glare—a study into glare recovery time with night driving spectacles. *Br. J. Physiol. Opt.*, **22**, 153–64.

Phillips, A.J. and Rutstein, A. (1967). Amber night driving spectacles. A further study. *Br. J. Physiol. Optics.*, **24**, 161–205.

Rackoff, N. (1974). An investigation of age related changes in drivers visual search patterns and driving performance and the relation of tests of basic functional capacities. PhD Dissertation. The Ohio State University, Columbus, Ohio.

Rackoff, N.J. and Mourant, R.R. (1979). Driving performance in the elderly. *Accid. Annal. Prev.*, **11**, 247–53.

Richards, O.W. (1953). Yellow glasses fail to improve seeing at night driving luminances. *Highway Research Abstracts*, **23**, 32–6.

Road Accidents Great Britain (1989). *The casualty report.* Department of Transport, HMSO, London.

Road Research Laboratory (1963). *Research on road safety.* HMSO, London.

Road Vehicle Lighting Regulations (1989). *Statutory instrument SI: 1989/1796.*, HMSO, London.

Sabey, B.E. and Johnson, H.D. (1973). *Road lighting and accidents: before and after studies on trunk road sites. Transport and Road Research Laboratory. Report No. LR586.* Transport and Road Research Laboratory, Crowthorne, Berkshire.

Statutory Instrument No. 1378 (1987). *Road traffic. Motor vehicles (driving licenses) regulations.* HMSO, London.

Staughton, G.C. and Storie, V.J. (1977). *Methodology of an in-depth accident investigation survey. Transport and Road Research Laboratory. Report No. LR762.* Transport and Road Research Laboratory, Crowthorne, Berkshire.

Sturgis, S.P. and Osgood, D.J. (1982). Effects of glare and background luminance on visual acuity and contrast sensitivity: implications for driver night vision testing. *Human Factors*, **24**, 347–50.

Taylor, J.F. (1987). Vision and driving. *Ophthal. Physiol.* Opt., **7**, 187–9.

Transport and Road Research Laboratory, (1980). *Gap acceptance and traffic conflict simulation as a measure of risk, Report No. SR 776.* Crowthorne, Berkshire.

Wolf, E., McFarland, R.A., and Zigler, M. (1960). Influence of tinted windshield glass on five visual functions. *Highway Research Board Bulletin*, **255**, 30–46.

Appendix A: Guidelines for the suitability of colour vision defects for certain occupations

(Courtesy of J. Voke and Keeler Ltd. 1980)

Jobs, careers, and industries where defective colour vision is a handicap and in which important consequences might result from errors of colour judgement

Air traffic controller

Buyers—textile, yarns, tobacco, food, e.g. fruit, cocoa, timber

Car body resprayer, retoucher

Cartographer

Ceramics—painter/decorater of pottery

Ceramics—inspector (quality control)

Chemist and chemicals:
laboratory analysis
food chemist
teacher of chemistry
manufacturer of chemicals and polishes and oils

Colour printer, etcher, retoucher

Colour photographer

Colour TV technician

Coloured pencils/chalks/paints manufacturing

Colourist/colour matcher in paints, paper, pigments, inks, dyes, wallpaper

Cotton grader

Coroner

Forensic scientist

Market gardener, e.g. fruit

Meat inspector

Oil refining

Paint maker and distributor

Paper making

Pharmacist

Plastics

Restorer of painting/works of art

Safety officer

Tanner

Tobacco grader

Jobs and careers where good vision is desirable but in which defective colour vision would not necessarily cause a handicap

Accountant

Anaesthetist

Architect

Artist—graphic, commercial, advertising

Auctioneer

Barmaid/barman

Bacteriologist

Baker

Beautician

Botanist

Brewer

Builder/bricklayer

Buyer—textiles, yarn, tobacco, food, e.g. fruit, cocoa, timber

Carpenter

Carpet/lino fitter/planner

Chiropodist

Clothes designer

Cook or chef

Confectioner

Cosmetics director (stage, film, TV)

Dental surgeon and technician

Draughtsman

Dressmaker

Driving instructor

Driver in public services, e.g. bus

Engineer (various)

Farmer

Fishmonger

Florist

Forester

Furrier

Gardener and landscape gardener

Geologist

Gemmologist, e.g. setting stones, diamond grader

Grocer

Hairdresser

Horticulturist

Illuminating engineer

Interior decorator/designer/planner

Jeweller

Librarian

Lighting director (state/film TV)

Manicurist

Metallurgist

Milliner

Miner

Nurse

Optometrist/ophthalmologist

Osteopath

Painter

Pharmacist assistant (counter service)

Physician

Physiotherapist

Post Office counter assistant

Potter

Salesman/woman (fabrics, drapery, yarns, wool, carperts) garments/footwear china and glass linen cosmetics/toiletries jewellery confectioner stationer storekeeper

Shoe repairer

Surgeon

Tanner

Tailor

Telephone switchboard operator

Theatre/stage props manager

Veterinary surgeon

Waiter

Zoologist

Jobs and careers requiring perfect colour vision

Armed forces—certain grades

Civil aviation

Colour matcher in dyeing, textiles, paints, inks, coloured paper, ceramics, cosmetics

Carpet darner/inspector, spinner, weaver, bobbin winder

Electrical work:
  electrician
  electronics technician
  colour TV mechanic
  motor mechanic
  telephone installer

Navigation—pilot, fisherman, railways

Police—certain grades

Radio—telegraphy

Appendix B: List of some of the suppliers of vision screeners

Model	Supplier

Essilor:
  Ergovision
  Visiotest
  Scolatest
	Central Safety Equipment Ltd,
	1 Myring Drive,
	Sutton Coldfield,
	West Midlands B75 7RZ, UK

Titmus II Vision Tester	Norville Optical Co. Ltd, Magdala Road, Gloucester GL1 4DG, UK
	Parmelee Ltd, Middlemore Lane West, Aldridge, Walsall, WS9 8DZ, UK
	Bolle (UK) Ltd, Brunel Close, Ebblake Industrial Estate, Verwood, Dorset BH31 6BA, UK
R10 (drivers) R11 (children) R12 (industrial)	Rodenstock (UK) Ltd, Springhead Road, Northfleet, Kent DA11 6HJ, UK
Topcon Screenoscope SS-3	Tinsley Medical Instruments, 275 King Henry's Drive, New Addington, Croydon, Surrey, CR0 0AE, UK
Keystone VS-2 DVS-11 Driver Vision Screen	Warwick-Evans Optical Co. Ltd, 22 Palace Road, Bounds Green, London NII 2PS, UK
Optec 2000	Grafton Optical Co. Ltd, 155–159 Queens Road, Watford, Herts WD1 2QH, UK
Binoptometer	Oculus Optikgerate GmbH, Munchholzhauser Straße 29, Dutenhofen, D-6330 Wetzlar 17, Germany

Appendix C: Shade numbers of filters recommended for welding BS 679 (EN 169)

Table: Shade numbers of filters to be used during gas welding and brazing

Flow rates q of acetylene	Type of operation	
	Welding and brazing of heavy metals	Welding with emissive fluxes (notably light alloys)
(L/h)		
$q \leq 70$	4	4F
$70 < q \leq 200$	5	5F
$200 < q \leq 800$	6	6F
$800 < q$	7	7F

NOTE 1. According to the conditions of use, the next greater or the next smaller shade number can be used.
NOTE 2. The term 'heavy metals' applies to steels, alloy steels, copper and its alloys, etc.

NB. EN 169 uses 'a' to denote welding with flux instead of 'F'.

Table: Shade numbers of filters to be used during oxygen cutting

Flow rate q of oxygen	Shade no.
(L/h)	
$900 \leq q \leq 2000$	5
$2000 < q \leq 4000$	6
$4000 < q \leq 8000$	7

NOTE. According to the conditions of use, the next greater or the next smaller shade number can be used.

Table: Shade numbers of filters recommended for use during arc welding

Welding process or related techniques	Current, A								
	0.5–20	20–40	40–80	80–125	125–225	225–350	350–450	450–500	
Covered electrodes	*(not used)*	9	10	11	11	12	13	14	
MIG on heavy metals	*(not used)*	*(not used)*	*(not used)*	10	11	12	13	14	
MIG on light alloys	*(not used)*	*(not used)*	*(not used)*	10	11	12	13	14–15	
TIG on all metals and alloys	*(not used)*	9	10	11	12	13–14	*(not used)*	*(not used)*	
MAG	*(not used)*	*(not used)*	10	11	12	13	14	15	
Air–arc cutting	*(not used)*	*(not used)*	*(not used)*	*(not used)*	10	11–12	13–14	15	
Plasma arcwelding	*(not used)*	*(not used)*	11	11	12	13	*(not used)*	*(not used)*	
Micro-plasma arc welding	4 5 6 7 8 9 10	11	12	12	13	14	14	15	

Current scale (A): 0.5 1 2.5 5 10 15 20 30 40 60 80 100 125 150 175 200 225 250 270 300 350 400 450 500

NOTE 1. According to the conditions of use, the next greater or the next smaller shade number can be used.

NOTE 2. The term 'heavy metals' applies to steels, alloy steels, copper and its alloys, etc.

NOTE 3. The hatched parts of the table indicate conditions where welding is not normally employed.

NOTE 4. The terms in column 1 are used in accordance with BS 499 : Part 1:
  (a) MIG refers to metal-arc welding with an inert gas shield;
  (b) MAG refers to metal-arc welding with a non-inert gas shield;
  (c) TIG refers to tungsten-arc welding with an inert gas shield;
  (d) air-arc cutting corresponds to the use of a carbon electrode and a jet of compressed air to remove the molten metal;
  (e) covered electrode refers to a consumable electrode having a covering of flux or other material.

Appendix D: Photometric units and the conversion factors necessary to change them to SI units

Quantity	Unit	Dimensions	Conversion factor
Illuminance	Lux	lumen/metre^2	1.0
	Metre candle	lumen/metre^2	1.0
SI unit = Lux	Phot	lumen/centimetre^2	10,000.0
	Footcandle	lumen/foot^2	10.76
Luminance	Nit	Candela/metre^2	1.0
	Stilb	candela/centimetre^2	10,000.0
SI unit =	Apostilb	lumen/metere^2	0.32
Candela/metre^2	Lambert	lumen/centimetre^2	3,183.0
	Footlambert	lumen/foot^2	3.43

Appendix E: Vision standards for various occupations

Vehicle drivers

Private motorists

The Motor Vehicles (Driving Licences) Regulations 1987 (SI No. 1378). The person should be able to read in good daylight (with the aid of glasses or contact lenses if worn) a number plate at a distance of 20.5 metres containing letters and figures 79.4 mm high.

A driving licence may not be granted to a person who suffers from some other disability likely to cause the driving of a vehicle to be a source of danger. The standards used are those detailed in the Medical Aspects of Fitness to Drive. The recommendations given include a horizontal visual field of not less than 120 degrees, no substantial binocular field loss especially in the lower quadrants, no diplopia, no marked degree of night vision defect. A monocular person may drive providing the visual acuity and visual field are adequate. An adaptation period may be required after the loss of an eye. The driver should report to the Licensing Centre if the above requirements can not be met.

Large Goods and Passenger Carrying Vehicles

The person should have a visual acuity (with glasses or contact lenses) of at least 6/9 in the better eye and 6/12 in the worst eye. The uncorrected vision in each eye should be 3/60 or better.

For renewal of a licence, which was held prior to 1 January 1983 and still held on 1 April 1991, the visual acuity should be at least 6/12 in the better eye and at least 6/36 in the worse eye. If the driver needs to wear glasses or contact lenses, the uncorrected acuity must be not less than 3/60 in each eye.

A spare pair of spectacles should be carried by those who have an uncorrected vision of 6/18 or worse. Visual fields should be tested by the hand confrontation test, which should be full and show no contraction. Any patholgical field defects, insuperable diplopia or monocular vision (except for some renewals) should rule out the driving of large goods and passenger carrying vehicles.

The driver's licence should be renewed at 45 or every 5 years, which ever is the longer. From the age of 45 renewals are every 5 years and from the age of 65 they are annually.

Civil Aviation Authority

The standards required for professional pilots and air traffic controllers are:

1. There shall be no acute or chronic disease in either eye or adnexa.
2. The visual fields must be normal.
3. A visual acuity of at least 6/9 in each eye (with or without glasses). The unaided vision must not be less than 6/60 or the refractive error must not exceed + or − 3.00 dioptres (equivalent sphere error). The medical certificate shall bear an endorsement noting the requirement to wear correcting lenses.
4. At the initial examination, any degree of heterophoria in excess of 8 prism dioptres exophoria, 6 prism dioptres esophoria or 1.5 prism dioptres hyperphoria will require further evaluation.
5. Candidates should be able to read N5 or its equivalent at a distance between 30–50 cm with each eye (with or without glasses). It is also required that N14 print should be read at 100 cm. The medical certificate should bear an endorsement noting the requirement to have available correcting glasses for near vision purposes.
6. Contact lenses may be worn by professional pilots subject to certain conditions. Full details can be obtained from the CAA Medical Department, but in the main applicants must have worn the contact lenses for several hours a day (the duration of a working day at least) for at least three months. Details of the lenses and a full ophthalmic report should be submitted.
7. The candidate should have normal colour vision perception as tested by Ishihara Pseudo-Isochromatic plates in good daylight or alternatively be able to recognise colours of signal red, signal green and white using the Holmes Wright Lantern as standard at a distance of 20 feet.

The standards for student and private pilots are:

1. There shall be no acute or chronic disease in either eye or adnexa.
2. The visual fields must be normal.
3. A visual acuity of at least 6/12 in each eye (with or without glasses). The unaided vision must be at least 6/60 and the refractive error must not exceed + or −5 dioptres (equivalent spherical error). Errors in excess of 5 but not exceeding 8 dioptres may be accepted provided that an ophthalmologist's assessment confirms that the retinae and fundi are healthy.

4. Any degree of heterophoria found in the test should be noted in the candidate's medical record.

5. The candidate shall be required to have accommodation that permits the reading of the Faculty of Ophthalmologists Reading Chart N5 or its equivalent at a distance between 30 and 50 cm with each eye, with or without glasses.

    The medical certificate will bear endorsement noting the requirement to have available correcting glasses for near vision purposes.

6. The wearing of contact lenses is permitted subject to certain conditions.

7. Monocular cases should be referred directly to the Civil Aviation Authority Medical Department, CAA House, 45/49 Kingsway, London, WC2B 6TE.

8. The candidate shall have normal colour vision perception as tested by Ishihara Pseudo-Isochromatic plates in good daylight or, alternatively, shall be able to recognize accurately the colours of red, green and white, using the Giles Archer or Holmes Wright lanterns, at a distance of 20 feet.

Further details can be obtained from the CAA, Aviation House, South Area, Gatwick Airport, Gatwick, W. Sussex RH6 0YR.

Visual display unit operators

AOP recommendations on the visual standards for VDU operators.

1. The ability to read N6 at a distance of 0.66 metre down to 0.33 metre.

2. Monocular or good binocular vision. Near phorias over 1/2 prism dioptre vertical or 2 prism dioptre esophoria and 8 prism dioptres exophoria at working distance are contraindicated and should be corrected unless well compensated or deep suppression is present.

3. No central (20 degrees) field defects in the dominant eye.

4. Near point of convergence normal.

5. Clear ocular media examined by ophthalmoscopy and slit lamp. The above recommendations are intended to increase the level of operator comfort, and therefore efficiency, but failure to achieve the standard does not exclude a person from working with a VDU.

For other vision standards, including the Armed Forces, see the AOP Handbook.

The above standards are reproduced by kind permission of the Controller of HMSO, The Association of Optometrists and The Civil Aviation Authorities.

Appendix F: The Personal Protective Equipment Regulations 1992

The Personal Protective Equipment Regulations 1992 have been introduced as amendments to The Health and Safety at Work etc. Act 1974. Hence most of the older legislation regarding personal protective equipment has been revoked including The Protection of Eyes Regulations 1974.

The Management of Health and Safety at Work Regulations 1992 requires the employers to identify and assess the risks to health and safety present in the workplace. Then, the most appropriate method of reducing the risks to an acceptable level can be decided. The provision of personal protective equipment (PPE) should be viewed as a last resort. The risks should be controlled by other means wherever possible. For example, a fixed shield placed in front of a grinding wheel could provide protection against flying particles instead of eye-protectors. The PPE Regulations cover protective clothing, e.g. gloves and footwear and protective equipment, e.g. life jackets and eye-protectors. It is the responsibility of employers to make sure that any PPE supplied to their employees is appropriate for the risks concerned. As far as eye-protectors are concerned the employer (and self-employed) must identify the hazard/s present, such as chemicals or flying particles, and then assess the degree of risk, for example the probable size and velocity of any flying particles. Once the hazard has been assessed a suitable type of PPE can be selected from the range of 'CE' marked equipment. The PPE should fit correctly, after adjustment if necessary. Where more than one type of PPE is necessary, they should be compatible and still be effective against the risks.

The PPE should be maintained so that it continues to provide the protection required. This may include cleaning, examination, replacement, repair and testing. A stock of spare parts, when appropriate, should be made available to the wearers. The regulations also require employers to provide suitable information, instruction and training so that effective use of PPE will be made by the employees. They must be trained in the correct use of the equipment, how to correctly fit and wear it and store it.

The employees also have a responsibility to wear PPE provided and to report any loss or defect to the employer as soon as possible.

Any PPE supplied for use at work must comply with the UK legislation implementing the European Community directives concerning design or manufacture with regard to health and safety. These are listed in Schedule 1 of the Regulations. The PPE (Safety) Regulations require that most PPE supplied for use at work must be certified by an independent inspection body. If the PPE conforms to the basic safety requirements then a certificate of conformity will be issued and the manufacturer is then able to mark the product with 'CE'. Once these regulations are in force it will be illegal for suppliers to sell PPE unless it is 'CE' marked.

The Health and Safety Executive has compiled a document to provide guidance on the PPE regulations. It states each regulation and then a section on guidance is given. Part 1 deals with major issues of the regulations and part 2 gives advice on the selection, use and maintenance of PPE. This document is very useful and should be consulted as the above is only an outline. The actual regulations should be consulted by employers.

Personal Protective Equipment Regulations 1992. Guidance on Regulations L25 is available from HMSO, mail order telephone 071 873 9090 or telefax 071 873 0011.

Glossary of terms

The majority of these terms are taken from *The dictionary of optometry*, (2nd edn), by kind permission of M. Millodot and Butterworth–Heinemann Ltd.

Accommodation. Adjustment of the dioptric power of the eye. It is generally involuntary and is made to see objects clearly at any distance. In man, this adjustment is brought about by a change in the shape of the crystalline lens.

accommodation, amplitude of. The maximum amount of accommodation that one eye can exert. It is expressed in dioptres(D), as the difference between the far point and the near point, measured with respect to the spectacle plane, the corneal apex, or some other reference point. The amplitude of accommodation declines from about 14 D at age 10 to about 0.5 D at age 60 (although the measured value is usually higher due to the depth of focus of the eye).

accommodation, range of. The linear distance between the far point and the near point.

acuity, dynamic. Capacity to see moving objects distinctly. Also referred to as kinetic acuity.

acuity, visual. Capacity for seeing the details of an object distinctly. Quantitatively, it is represented in two ways:

1. As the reciprocal of the minimum angle of resolution (in minutes of arc). This is the resolution visual acuity.
2. As the Snellen fraction. This is measured using letters or **Landolt rings,** or equivalent objects.

Average clinical visual acuity varies between 6/4 and 6/6 (or 20/15 and 20/20 in feet). Visual acuity varies with the region of the retina (being maximum at the foveola), with general illumination, contrast, colour and type of test, time of exposure, the refractive error of the eye, etc.

Static visual acuity is the capacity for seeing distinctly the details of a stationary target.

adaptation, dark. Adjustment of the eye (particularly the retinal pigments but also the pupil) such that, after observation in the dark, the sensitivity to light is greatly increased, i.e. the threshold response to light is decreased. This is a much slower process than light adaptation.

adaptation, light. Adjustment of the eye (particularly the retinal pigments but also the pupil), such that after observation of a bright field, the sensitivity to light is diminished, i.e. the threshold of luminance is increased.

amblyopia. A condition characterized by low visual acuity without any apparent lesion of the eye or proven disorder in the visual pathway that is not correctable by optical means.

ametropia. Anomaly of the refractive state of the eye in which, with relaxed accommodation, the image of objects at infinity is not formed on the retina. Thus vision may be blurred. The ametropias are: **astigmatism**, **hypermetropia**, and **myopia**. The absence of ametropia is called **emmetropia**.

anisometropia. Condition in which the refractive state of a pair of eyes differs. Therefore one eye requires a lens power that is different to that of the other eye.

asthenopia. Term used to describe any symptoms associated with the use of the eyes. The causes of asthenopia are numerous: sustained near vision, either when the accommodation amplitude is low or hypermetropia is uncorrected (accommodative asthenopia), aniseikonia (aniseikonic asthenopia), astigmatism (astigmatic asthenopia), pain in the eye (asthenopia dolens), heterophoria (heterophoric asthenopia), ocular inflammation (asthenopia irritans), hysteria (nervous asthenopia), uncorrected presbyopia (presbyopic asthenopia), improper illumination (photogenous asthenopia), or retinal disease (retinal asthenopia).

astigmatism. A condition of refraction in which the image of a point object is not a single point but two mutually perpendicular lines at different distances from the optical system. The two focal lines are perpendicular to each other. In the eye, astigmatism is a refractive error that is generally caused by one or several toroidal shapes of the refracting surfaces, or by the obliquity of the light entering the eye, but it can also develop as a result of a subluxation of the lens or as a result of diabetes, cataract, or trauma (acquired astigmatism).

candela. A measure of luminous intensity, which is the power of a source or illuminated surface to emit light in a given direction. One candela is equal to one lumen per steradian.

cataract. Partial or complete loss of transparency of the crystalline lens substance or its capsule. Cataract may occur as a result of age, trauma, systemic disease (e.g. diabetes), ocular disease (e.g. anterior uveitis), high myopia, long-term steroid therapy, excessive exposure to IR and UV light, heredity, and maternal infections, (Down syndrome, etc.). The main symptom is a gradual loss of vision, often described as 'misty'.

Some patients may also notice transient monocular diplopia, others fixed spots (not floaters) in the visual field, and others better vision in dim illumination.

chart, Snellen. A visual acuity test using a graduated series of Snellen letters (or Snellen test types) in which the limbs and the spaces between them subtend an angle of one min of arc at specified distances. The letters are usually constructed so that they are five units high and four units wide, although some charts use letters which fit within a square subtending 5 min of arc at that distance.

CIE. Abbreviation for Commission Internationale de l'Eclairage.

colour, confusion. Colours that are confused by a dichromat. The colours confused by a deuteranope, a protanope, and a tritanope are not the same. A deuteranope will confuse reds, greens, and greys, whereas a protanope will confuse reds, orange, blue–greens, and greys.

convergence. 1. Movement of the eyes turning inwards or towards each other. 2. Characteristic of a pencil of light rays directed towards a real image point.

convergence insufficiency. An inability to converge, or to maintain convergence, usually associated with a high exophoria at near and a relatively orthophoric condition at distance. It results in complaints of fatigue, or even diplopia, due to the inability to maintain (and sometimes even to obtain) adequate convergence for prolonged close work.

convergence, near point of. The nearest point where the lines of sight intersect when the eyes converge to the maximum. This point is normally about 8 cm from the spectacle plane. If further away, the patient may have convergence insufficiency.

depth perception. See **perception, depth**.

differential threshold. The smallest difference between two stimuli presented simultaneously that gives rise to a perceived difference in sensation. The difference may be related to brightness, but also to colour and specifically to either saturation (whilst hue is kept constant) or hue (whilst saturation is kept constant). The differential threshold of luminance is equal to about 1 per cent photopic vision.

dioptre. (Symbol D) A unit indicating the refractive power of a lens or of an optical system. It is equal to the product of the refractive index in the image space and the reciprocal of the focal length in metres. Thus a lens with a focal length (in air) of 1 m has a power of 1 D, one with a focal length of 1/2 m, has a power of 2 D, etc.

diplopia. The condition in which a single object is seen as two rather than one. This is usually due to images not stimulating corresponding retinal areas in each of a pair of eyes.

disability glare. See **glare, disability**.

discomfort glare. See **glare, discomfort**.

disparity, retinal (fixation). Binocular vision in which the retinal image in each eye does not quite fall on corresponding retinal points. As the discrepancy is very small it is not experienced as diplopia. However, in some cases, it can cause symptoms of eye strain.

dispersion. The separation of light into its monochromatic components.

divergence. 1. Movement of the eyes turning away from each other so that the lines of sight intersect behind the eyes. 2. Characteristic of a pencil of light rays, as when emanating from a point source.

emmetropia. Refractive condition of the eye in which distant objects are focused on the retina, when accommodation is relaxed. This is the ideal refractive state of the eye.

esophoria. Turning of the eye inward when binocular vision is interrupted.

esotropia (convergent strabismus). Strabismus in which the deviating eye turns inwards. This is the most common type of strabismus in children.

exophoria. Turning of the eye outwards when binocular vision is interrupted.

exotropia (divergent strabismus). Strabismus in which the deviating eye turns outwards.

fatigue, visual. Feeling of a diminuition in visual performance, which is not necessarily produced by an excessive use of the eyes. However, there does not seem to be concrete objective proof of a reduction in visual aptitude (e.g. **visual acuity**) accompanying visual fatigue.

field, visual. The extent of space in which objects are visible to an eye in a given position. The visual field extends to approximately 100 ° temporally, 60 ° nasally, 65 ° superiorly and 75 ° inferiorly. The visual field can be measured either monocularly or binocularly. In the latter case its extent is much larger, especially in the horizontal plane.

filter. See **lens, absorptive**.

fusion. The process by which the retinal images from each eye are perceived as a single percept. In normal binocular vision this occurs when each eye is directed at the object and the image falls on corresponding retinal points.

glare. A visual condition in which the observer feels discomfort and/or exhibits a lower performance in visual tests (e.g. visual acuity or contrast sensitivity). This is produced by a relatively bright source of light (called the glare source) within the visual field. A given bright light may or may not produce glare, depending upon the location, the intensity of the light source, the background luminance, the state of adaptation of the eye, and the clarity of the media of the eye.

glare, disability. Glare that reduces visual performance without necessarily causing discomfort.

glare, discomfort. Glare that produces discomfort without necessarily interfering with visual performance.

heterophoria. The condition where the lines of sight of a pair of eyes do not meet at the fixation point when binocular vision is interrupted. The deviation can take various forms according to its relative direction, e.g. esophoria, exophoria, hyperphoria, hypophoria.

heterotropia (strabismus, squint). The condition in which the lines of sight of the two eyes are not directed towards the same fixation point when the subject is actively fixating an object. Thus, the image of the fixation point is not formed on the fovea of the deviating eye and there may be diplopia. In most cases the diplopic image is suppressed and vision is essentially monocular.

hyper(metr)opia. Refraction condition of the eye in which distant objects are focused behind the retina when the accommodation is relaxed; thus, vision is blurred. In hypermetropia, the point conjugate with the retina, that is the far point of the eye, is located behind the eye.

hyperphoria. The tendency for the line of sight of one eye to deviate upwards relative to that of the other eye, when binocular vision is interrupted. If the deviation tends to be downwards relative to the other eye, or if the other eye in hyperphoria is used as a reference, the condition is called hypophoria.

hypertropia. Strabismus in which one eye is directed to the fixation point whilst the other is directed upwards (right or left hypertropia). If one eye fixates whilst the other is directed downwards the condition is called hypotropia (right or left hypotropia).

illuminants, CIE standard. The colorimetric illuminants A, B, C, and D65 defined by the CIE in terms of relative spectral energy (power distribution): standard illuminant A representing the full radiator at T = 2854 K; standard illuminant B representing direct sunlight with a correlated colour temperature of T = 4874 K; standard illuminant C representing daylight with a correlated colour temperature of T = 6774 K; standard illuminant D representing daylight with a correlated colour temperaure of T = 6504 K (CIE).

illumination. Quotient of the luminous flux incident on an element of surface by the area of that element of surface. Symbol: E. The units are lux (lx) or footcandles.

interpupillary distance. The distance between the centres of the pupils of the eyes. It usually refers to the eyes fixating at infinity, otherwise reference must be made to the fixation distance (e.g. near interpupillary distance). The average interpupillary distance for men is about 64 mm and for women about 62 mm.

Kelvin. The Kelvin (K) unit of thermodynamic temperature, is the fraction 1/273.16 of the thermodynamic temperature of the triple point of water.

Landolt ring. A test object used for measuring visual acuity consisting of an incomplete ring resembling the letter C. The width of the break and of the ring are each one-fifth of its overall diameter. The subject must indicate where the break is located. The mimimum angle of resolution corresponds to the angular subtense of the just noticeable break, at the eye.

laser. An intense luminous source of coherent and monochromatic light. The term is an acronym for Light Amplification by Stimulated Emission of Radiation.

lens, absorptive. A (tinted) lens that absorbs a proportion of the incident radiation. Some lenses absorb in the infra-red region of the spectrum, others absorb in the ultraviolet region and others absorb more or less equally throughout, or selectively in, the visible spectrum.

lens, afocal. A lens of zero power.

lens, laminated. A lens consisting of a thin layer of plastic (e.g. cellulose acetate) cemented between two layers of glass. Such a lens provides mechanical protection for the eye because in case of breakage the glass pieces remain attached to the plastics layer.

lens, safety. 1. A lens made of safety glass. 2. A general term referring to any lens that protects the eyes against injury due to impact. It is more resistant to fracture and less likely to splinter than an ordinary glass lens. Examples: plastics lenses (especially polycarbonate), toughened lenses, laminated lenses. Plastics lenses have the greatest impact resistance of all these lenses.

lens, single-vision. An ophthalmic lens providing a correction for one viewing distance.

lens, toughened. A lens made of glass that has been thermally or chemically strengthened.

lens, trifocal. A multifocal lens consisting of three portions of different focal powers, usually for distance, intermediate, and near vision.

lens, varifocal; progressive. A spectacle lens having a gradual and progressive change in power either over the whole lens or over a region intermediate between areas of uniform power. This lens is used to correct presbyopia. There are several types, which are known by their tradenames (e.g. Progressive R, Truvision, Varilux).

light. Electromagnetic vibration capable of stimulating the receptors of the retina and producing a visual sensation. The radiations that give rise to the sensation of vision are comprised within the wavelength band 380–760 nm. This band is called the visible spectrum. The borders of this band are not precise, but beyond these radiations the visual efficacy of any wavelength becomes very low indeed (less than 10^{-5}). For an older subject, the lower boundary of the visible spectrum is closer to 420 nm than 380 nm.

line of sight. Line joining the point of fixation to the centre of the entrance pupil of the eye. The entrance pupil is what one sees when looking at an eye and is the image of the iris aperture formed by the cornea.

lumen. SI unit of luminous flux. It is equal to the flux emitted within a unit solid angle of one steradian by a point source with a luminous intensity of one candela. Symbol: lm.

luminaire. An electric light fitting that distributes, filters, or transforms the light and includes all the accessory items of the fittings.

luminance. Photometric term characterizing the way in which a surface emits or reflects light in a given direction. It is equal to the luminous intensity measured in a given direction divided by the area of this surface projected on a perpendicular to the direction considered. Symbol: L. Units: candela per square metre (cd/m^2); footlambert; lambert.

luminous intensity. Quotient of the luminous flux leaving the source, propagated in an element of solid angle containing the given direction, by the element of solid angle. Symbol: I. Unit: candela (cd).

lux. SI unit of illumination. It is the illumination produced by a luminous flux of one lumen uniformly distributed over a surface area of one square metre. Symbol: lx.

mesopic. See **vision, mesopic**.

miosis. A condition in which the pupil is constricted.

myopia. Refractive condition of the eye in which distant objects are focused in front of the retina when the accommodation is relaxed. Thus distance vision is blurred. In myopia the point conjugate with the retina, i.e. the far point of the eye, is located at some finite distance in front of the eye.

nanometre. Unit of length equal to one-thousand-millionth of a metre (10 ångströms or 10^{-9} m). Abbreviation: nm.

ophthalmoscopy. Method of examination of the interior of the eye with an ophthalmoscope.

optometrist. A person licensed (or registered) to practice optometry (definition of the International Optometric and Optical League).

perception, depth. Perception of relative or absolute differences in distance of objects from the observer. Depth perception is more precise in binocular vision, but is possible in monocular vision using the following cues: interposition, relative position, relative size, linear perspective, textual gradient, aerial perspective, light and shade, shadow, and motion parallax.

photometer. An instrument for measuring the luminous intensity of a light source or a surface, by comparing it with a standard source. The comparison can be done either with the human eye or with a photoelectric cell.

photophobia. Ocular discomfort induced by bright lights.

photopic. See **vision, photopic**.

plastics. Various organic or synthetic materials (e.g. CR39, HEMA, polymethylmethacrylate, etc.), which can be transformed into solid shapes to make spectacle frames, contact lenses, ophthalmic lenses, etc. They can be made to have good optical surfaces, high light transmission and refractive indices, and dispersions corresponding to that of crown or flint glass.

presbyopia. A refractive condition in which the accommodative ability of the eye becomes insufficient for satisfactory near vision without the use of corrective plus lenses (called the addition). This condition generally occurs between the ages of 42 and 48 in people living in Europe and North American countries.

prism dioptre. A unit specifying the amount of deviation by an ophthalmic prism. One prism dioptre represents a deviation of 1 cm on a flat surface 1 m away from the prism.

refractive error. The dioptric power of the ametropia of the eye. It is equal to the reciprocal of the distance between the far point and the eye, in metres.

retinoscopy. The determination of the refractive state of the eye by means of a retinoscope.

refractive index. The ratio of the speed of light in a vacuum or in air, to the speed of light in a given medium (Symbol: n). The speed of light in a given medium depends upon the wave length of light and, consequently, the index varies accordingly. The index of refraction forms the basis of Snell's law, which quantitatively determines the deviation of light rays traversing a surface separating two media of different refractive indices.

scotoma. An area (of partial or complete) blindness surrounded by normal or relatively normal visual field.

scotopic. See vision, scotopic.

SI unit. The Système international d'Unités.

slit lamp. An instrument consisting of an illuminating system and a microscope. It can be used to examine the anterior segment of the eye. (Supplementary lenses are required to view the posterior segment.)

strabismus. See **heterotropia**.

threshold, absolute. The minimum luminance of a source that will produce a sensation of light. It varies with the state of dark adaptation, the retinal area stimulated, the type of stimulus, etc.

vision, colour. Vision in which the colour sense is experienced.

vision, mesopic. Vision at intermediate levels between photopic and scotopic vision and corresponds to luminances ranging from 10^{-3} to 10 cd/m^2.

vision, photopic. Vision at high levels of luminance (above 10 cd/m^2) and resulting from the functioning of the cones.

vision, scotopic. Vision at low levels of luminance, below about 10^{-3} cd/m^2 and resulting from the functioning of the rods.

visual acuity. See **acuity, visual**.

visual fatigue. See **fatigue, visual**.

visual field. See **field, visual**.

Index